Resident's Guide to

Clinical
Psychiatry

The Resident Editorial Board

Resident's Guide to

Clinical Psychiatry

Lauren B. Marangell, M.D.

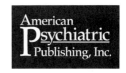

Washington, DC
London, England

DSM-IV-TR criteria tables throughout this book are reprinted from American Psychiatric Association: *Diagnostic and Statistical Manual of Mental Disorders, 4th Edition, Text Revision.* Washington, DC, American Psychiatric Association, 2000. Used with permission.

Manufactured in the United States of America on acid-free paper
12   11   10   09   08   5   4   3   2   1
First Edition

Typeset in Adobe's Palatino and Frutiger

American Psychiatric Publishing, Inc.
1000 Wilson Boulevard
Arlington, VA 22209-3901
www.appi.org

Library of Congress Cataloging-in-Publication Data
Marangell, Lauren B., 1961–
   Resident's guide to clinical psychiatry / by Lauren B. Marangell.—1st ed.
     p. ; cm.
   Includes bibliographical references and index.
   ISBN 978-1-58562-324-2 (alk. paper)
   1. Psychiatry—Handbooks, manuals, etc. 2. Residents (Medicine)—Handbooks, manuals, etc. I. American Psychiatric Publishing. II. Title.
[DNLM:1. Mental Disorders—therapy. WM140 M311r 2009]
RC456.M365 2009
616.89—dc22

                                           2008030966

British Library Cataloguing in Publication Data
A CIP record is available from the British Library.

Contents

Disclosure of Competing Interests

In the past 3 years, Lauren B. Marangell, M.D., has received grant and research support from Bristol-Myers Squibb Company, Eli Lilly and Company, Cyberonics, Neuronetics, the National Institute of Mental Health, the Stanley Foundation, NARSAD, the American Foundation for Suicide Prevention, Aspect Medical Systems, and Sanofi Aventis. She has also worked as a consultant for, or received honoraria from, Eli Lilly and Company, GlaxoSmithKline, Cyberonics, Pfizer, Medtronics, Forest, Aspect Medical Systems, Novartis, and Sepracor.

Dr. Marangell's work on *Resident's Guide to Clinical Psychiatry* was submitted for publication prior to beginning her full time position as a Distinguished Scholar with Eli Lilly and Company. The views expressed herein are hers alone, and not necessarily those of Eli Lilly and Company.

Foreword

It gives us great pleasure to write the preface to this excellent addition to the American Psychiatric Publishing (APPI) portfolio of books. We have worked with Dr. Lauren Marangell for many years in a number of educational, clinical, and research capacities and feel privileged to contribute to this text. Dr. Marangell is a psychopharmacologist with an outstanding research background. She trained in the Biological Psychiatry Branch of the National Institute of Mental Health. In1994, she moved to Baylor College of Medicine, where she founded and directed the Mood Disorders Center of the Menninger Department of Psychiatry and Behavioral Sciences. Recently she relinquished her position at Baylor College of Medicine to assume a research position at the Eli Lilly Company.

For a number of years, APPI has planned to publish a resident handbook to clinical psychiatry. We wanted an evidence-based, clinically-oriented guide that could fit into the lab coat of a psychiatry resident or medical student—a book they could consult frequently and conveniently during their clinical rotations. At the same time, APPI desired to craft a psychiatry guide that is concise, yet sufficiently comprehensive to be useful for residents training in psychiatry, primary care specialties, and clinical neuroscience-related specialties during all stages of their specialty training. Dr. Marangell, who was perennially among the most popular and effective educators for medical students and psychiatry residents during her many years on the Baylor faculty, as well as at national and international forums, was our first choice to meet our goals for *Resident's Guide to Clinical Psychiatry* (the *Guide*).

The *Guide* opens with an excellent chapter on assessment and documentation. This includes such practical information as a sample psychiatric initial evaluation, sample admitting orders, and outlines of the physical examination and neurological examination, as well as examples of progress notes, informed consent, and a hospital discharge summary. This chapter contains a wealth of valuable information and suggested templates that residents can follow when assessing and documenting their treatment of patients.

The next nine chapters of the *Guide* focus on the most common (and disabling) psychiatric disorders that medical students and residents are most likely to encounter during their clinical rotations in psychiatry, including: psychotic disorders, mood disorders, anxiety disorders, personality disorders, sleep disorders, substance-related disorders, dementia, factitious disorders and somatoform disorders, and eating disorders. Each chapter includes brief epidemiologic information, diagnostic criteria, differential diagnosis, and treatment recommendations.

To complement the nine disorder-based chapters, Dr. Marangell includes chapters on major psychiatric rotations on which all residents and many medical students will be assigned. These chapters comprise consultation-liaison psychiatry, emergency psychiatry, and child and adolescent psychiatry. The focus of the consultation-liaison psychiatry is documentation, capacity for health care decision making, and the assessment and treatment of delirium and other psychiatric disorders most frequently encountered in the medical setting. The emergency psychiatry chapter places emphasis on the most common psychiatric emergencies that residents and students will encounter, including the assessment and management of the suicidal patient. Finally, the chapter on child and adolescent psychiatry reviews the disorders most commonly found in children and adolescents by general psychiatry resident, including: developmental disorders, attention-deficit/hyperactivity disorder, conduct disorder and oppositional/defiant disorder, Tourette's disorder, mental retardation, major depressive disorder and bipolar disorder.

The *Guide* continues with two excellent chapters on pharmacotherapy and psychotherapy and psychosocial treatments. With Dr. Marangell being a noted research scientist, educator, and clinician in the realm of psychopharmacology, these chapters are true gems in that they include just the right amount of information on the major psychiatric classes of psychotropic medication that residents will prescribe, such as antipsychotics, antidepressants, mood stabilizers, anti-anxiety medications, sedatives and hypnotics, stimulants, and cognitive enhancers. The author concludes her book with a discussion of device-based treatments, including electroconvulsive therapy, vagus nerve stimulation, transcranial magnetic stimulation, and deep brain stimulation. We believe that device-based interventions will become increasingly important components of the clinical armamentarium of psychiatrists in the near future. Finally, the *Guide* contains two excellent appendices—one featuring commonly used abbreviations, and another listing trade names of frequently prescribed psychiatric medications. Notwithstanding our preference for the use of generic appellations for psychiatric medications, many professionals and patients still utilize trade names for psychiatric agents; therefore, it is important for residents and medical students to be familiar with these for purposes of facile communication in the clinical setting.

In summary, we highly recommend *Resident's Guide to Clinical Psychiatry* to medical students, psychiatry residents, and physicians in clinical practice who seek a user-friendly, practical, and concise book for assessing and treating patients with psychiatric disorders. We intend to carry this book around with us during our clinical and teaching rounds in our respective medical centers and advise that you consider doing so, as well. We are deeply appreciative to Dr. Marangell for a job well done.

Robert E. Hales, M.D., M.B.A.
Sacramento, California

Stuart C. Yudofsky, M.D.
Houston, Texas

Acknowledgments

As with many modern textbooks, this work has benefited greatly from the work of a large number of people. Multiple APPI authors generously allowed tables they created to be reproduced for this text. Editor-in-Chief Robert E. Hales, M.D., M.B.A, and the APPI editorial staff are of unparalleled caliber and have greatly facilitated this project. Throughout my career at Baylor College of Medicine, Dr. Stuart C. Yudofsky and the faculty and residents of that fine institution have provided ongoing inspiration for me to improve psychiatric education wherever possible. Holly Zboyan, M.A., and Linda Barloon, R.N., both with our Mood Disorders Center at Baylor College of Medicine at the time, were of extraordinary help in preparing this text. The Resident Editorial Board, formulated to prepare this text, was invaluable in ensuring that the text remained germane to trainees and reflective of broad perspectives. This text also benefited from prior collaborations with Drs. James Martinez, Stuart C. Yudofsky, and Jonathan Silver. Finally, I wish to express my gratitude to Dr. Kimberly Monday, who has not only provided many years of encouragement, but also made significant contributions to the sleep disorders section.

1

Assessment and Documentation

Psychiatry, like all areas of medicine, relies on proper diagnosis. Diagnosis in psychiatry is typically presented as a five-axis system that allows for the integrated presentation of major psychiatric disorders and describes the dimensions of psychiatric illness: biological basis, maladaptive personality patterns, nonpsychiatric medical problems, life stressors, and overall functioning. Hence, the typical model is referred to as biopsychosocial. Written psychiatric evaluations and presentations in rounds should typically include all five axes. If not enough information is available, the diagnosis on an axis may be "deferred." This is often the case with personality disorders, which typically require a longer period of assessment for correct diagnosis.

The five axes included in the multiaxial classification are

- Axis I: clinical psychiatric disorders (list all, with reason for visit listed first) and other conditions that may be the focus of clinical attention;

- Axis II: personality disorders and mental retardation;

- Axis III: general medical conditions;

- Axis IV: psychosocial and environmental problems and stresses, such as difficulty in a significant relationship; and

- Axis V: Global Assessment of Functioning (GAF). Typically, GAF ratings are given for current level of functioning and highest level of functioning in the past year. The GAF scale and anchor points are shown in Table 1–1.

TABLE 1–1.   Global Assessment of Functioning (GAF)
Scale

Code   (Note: Use intermediate codes when appropriate, e.g., 45, 68, 72.)

100 **Superior functioning in a wide range of activities, life's**
| **problems never seem to get out of hand, is sought out by**
91   **others because of his or her many positive qualities. No**
symptoms.

90 **Absent or minimal symptoms** (e.g., mild anxiety before an
| exam), **good functioning in all areas, interested and**
81   **involved in a wide range of activities, socially effective,**
generally satisfied with life, no more than everyday
problems or concerns (e.g., an occasional argument with
family members).

80 **If symptoms are present, they are transient and**
| **expectable reactions to psychosocial stressors** (e.g.,
71   difficulty concentrating after family argument); **no more than**
slight impairment in social, occupational, or school
functioning (e.g., temporarily falling behind in schoolwork).

70 **Some mild symptoms** (e.g., depressed mood and mild
| insomnia) **OR some difficulty in social, occupational, or**
61   **school functioning** (e.g., occasional truancy, or theft within
the household), **but generally functioning pretty well, has**
some meaningful interpersonal relationships.

60 **Moderate symptoms** (e.g., flat affect and circumstantial
| speech, occasional panic attacks) **OR moderate difficulty in**
51   **social, occupational, or school functioning** (e.g., few
friends, conflicts with peers or co-workers).

50 **Serious symptoms** (e.g., suicidal ideation, severe obsessional
| rituals, frequent shoplifting) **OR any serious impairment in**
41   **social, occupational, or school functioning** (e.g., no
friends, unable to keep a job).

TABLE 1–1. Global Assessment of Functioning (GAF)
Scale *(continued)*

40 **Some impairment in reality testing or communication** (e.g.,
| speech is at times illogical, obscure, or irrelevant) **OR major**
31 **impairment in several areas, such as work or school,**
family relations, judgment, thinking, or mood (e.g.,
depressed man avoids friends, neglects family, and is unable to
work; child frequently beats up younger children, is defiant at
home, and is failing at school).

30 **Behavior is considerably influenced by delusions or**
| **hallucinations OR serious impairment in communication**
21 **or judgment** (e.g., sometimes incoherent, acts grossly
inappropriately, suicidal preoccupation) **OR inability to**
function in almost all areas (e.g., stays in bed all day; no job,
home, or friends).

20 **Some danger of hurting self or others** (e.g., suicide attempts
| without clear expectation of death; frequently violent; manic
11 excitement) **OR occasionally fails to maintain minimal**
personal hygiene (e.g., smears feces) **OR gross impairment**
in communication (e.g., largely incoherent or mute).

10 **Persistent danger of severely hurting self or others** (e.g.,
| recurrent violence) **OR persistent inability to maintain**
1 **minimal personal hygiene OR serious suicidal act with**
clear expectation of death.

0 **Inadequate information.**

Note. The rating of overall psychological functioning on a scale of 0–100 was
operationalized by Luborsky in the Health-Sickness Rating Scale (Luborsky L:
"Clinicians' Judgments of Mental Health." Archives of General Psychiatry 7:407–417,
1962). Spitzer and colleagues developed a revision of the Health-Sickness Rating Scale called the Global Assessment Scale (GAS) (Endicott J, Spitzer RL,
Fleiss JL, et al: *"The Global Assessment Scale: A Procedure for Measuring Overall
Severity of Psychiatric Disturbance." Archives of General Psychiatry* 33:766–771,
1976). A modified version of the GAS was included in DSM-III-R as the Global
Assessment of Functioning (GAF) Scale.
Source. Reprinted from American Psychiatric Association: *Diagnostic and Statistical Manual of Mental Disorders, 4th Edition, Text Revision.* Washington, DC,
American Psychiatric Association, 2000, p 34. Used with permission.

The Interview

General Guidelines

- *Establish rapport.* On meeting a new patient, it is essential to first put the patient at ease. For example, introduce yourself, ask whether the patient is comfortable, and explain that you are just going to talk for X amount of time, e.g., about 45 minutes.

- *Ensure safety first.* Although most psychiatric patients are no more violent than other patients, it is imperative to ensure your own safety at all times. If a patient is potentially dangerous, the door should remain open and you should sit near the door. Likewise, a patient may become more agitated if he or she feels trapped in a room, so it is ideal if both parties have easy access to the exit. You may also ask security staff to be present or outside the door if you believe the patient may become violent.

- *Reduce communication barriers.* For patients who are not proficient in English or for patients with limited hearing, use professional interpreters who are trained in mental health. Avoid using family members to serve as interpreters because this affects confidentiality and may lead to biased answers.

- *Speak with collateral sources.* Information from family members and friends is often very useful. Ask the patient for permission to interview others and protect privacy by asking questions in a way that does not reveal confidential information (e.g., asking if Mr. A has ever been violent, as opposed to telling the family that Mr. A mentioned that he has been violent). If there is concern for a patient's safety, collateral information may be obtained without the patient's consent, but it is still wise to inform the patient that you are doing this.

- *Consider time constraints.* Attend to the patient's most pressing concerns first. If a patient is agitated or unable to tolerate a prolonged interview, you may need to complete the assessment over several sessions. Prioritize issues that require urgent treatment.

Specific Techniques

Start with open-ended questions, such as "So what brought you here?" "How did this come about?" or "How can we help you?" Unless you are in an emergency setting, allow the patient to speak with minimal interruptions for 5–10 minutes. This will give you some of the factual information you need and allow you to observe the patient carefully. Watch for eye contact, distractibility, and abnormal movements. Do the patient's thoughts seem logical and coherent, or are they hard to follow? Does the patient seem suspicious or anxious? Is the patient's speech unusually rapid? Much of the mental status information comes from such observations.

After 5–10 minutes, start asking more detailed questions to gather the information you need to make the correct diagnosis.

It is sometimes necessary to interrupt or redirect patients during the interview. A useful phrase, gently stated, is " Mr. A, I know this [topic] is important and hopefully we will have time to come back to it, but right now I need you to tell me about [information you need]." If this happens repeatedly, it is often helpful to explain to the patient that you have only X amount of time (e.g., 1 hour), and in order to best help him or her, you need to get some specific information and you are sorry to have to interrupt.

It is important that at the end of the interview the patient feels heard and supported and understands what will happen next, even if this is as vague as "I am going to talk to the rest of the team, and we will come up with a plan. I will talk to you about that tomorrow." Finally, allow the patient time to ask questions before departing.

Components of the Complete Psychiatric Evaluation

General identifying information (ID): Include age, race, sex, marital status, and occupation.

Chief complaint: Cite the patient's stated reason for evaluation.

Source of information: List sources used in preparing the evaluation, such as interview with the patient, review of records, referral information, and interviews with family members.

History of present illness: Ask about symptom clusters that will rule in or rule out specific diagnoses. Keep an open mind so that you do not overlook possible diagnoses. Note both positive and negative pertinent symptoms. Questions specific to common presentations, such as psychosis, depression, and anxiety, are included in subsequent chapters of this book. Be sure to inquire about mood symptoms, psychotic symptoms, anxiety symptoms, and alcohol and substance dependence (see Table 1–2).

TABLE 1–2.   Normal or psychopathology?

NORMAL	PSYCHOPATHOLOGY (AXIS I)
Symptoms are transient	Symptoms occur nearly every day and persist for weeks or months
Functioning reasonably well at work, home, etc.	Impaired functioning at work, home, etc., *or* substantial subjective distress
Symptoms are not significantly different from the person's baseline emotional state	Symptoms differ markedly from person's usual state
Loved ones are not overly concerned	Loved ones are extremely concerned that the symptoms are abnormal
Most healthy people experience these symptoms at least occasionally	Most people rarely or never experience these symptoms (e.g., hearing voices)

Past psychiatric history: Document prior treatment and treaters, including hospitalizations, medications, suicide attempts, and history of violence.

Medications: Include dosages, patient response, duration of treatment, and side effects for current psychiatric medications, past psychiatric medications, and current nonpsychiatric medications. Be sure to note any nonpsychiatric medications that the patient is currently taking that might cause drug–drug interactions. Also ask about herbal preparations and supplements that the patient may be taking but not think of as "medication."

Allergies: Note whether patient has any known drug allergies.

Psychiatric review of systems: The review of systems should include the following areas:

- Depression
- Mania
- Psychosis
- Anxiety/panic

- Obsessions/compulsions
- Binge eating or anorexia
- Thoughts of harm to self or others (including self-harm without the intent to die)

Past medical history: It is imperative to rule out nonpsychiatric causes for psychiatric symptoms, such as endocrine or neurological disorders. In addition, note the presence of other medical problems that might influence drug selection, such as cardiac or hepatic disease. If the patient is female and of childbearing potential, note if the patient uses contraception and if the contraceptive method may influence drug selection.

Family history: Note family history of psychiatric disorders and suicide.

Social and developmental history: One technique for taking a social and developmental history is to walk through the patient's life. Typical questions include, "Where did you grow up? Did you have brothers or sisters? How was life for you then? How far did you go in school? What happened after that? When did get your first job?"

It is important to inquire about and document the following information:

- Current family relationships and supports
- Current living situation and functional status
- Any cultural, religious, or spiritual issues that may affect care
- Legal problems (current and past)
- History of abuse, when and by whom (sexual, physical, and/or emotional)
- Occupational history/status

Substance abuse history: Note the type of substance and the amount and frequency of substances used, history of withdrawal symptoms, and history of treatment for substance-related disorders.

Physical and neurological examination: A number of psychiatric symptoms may be due to an underlying medical disorder. As such, a medical and neurological evaluation is required for new patients. In addition, the use of certain medications may require monitoring physical parameters such as weight, waist circumference, and blood pressure, as discussed in later chapters of this guide. Table 1–3 presents selected elements of the physical examination and the significance of findings. Components of

TABLE 1–3.   Selected elements of the physical examination and the significance of findings

ELEMENTS	EXAMPLES OF POSSIBLE DIAGNOSES
General	
Appearance healthier than expected	Somatoform disorder
Fever	Infection or NMS
Blood pressure or pulse abnormalities	Withdrawal, thyroid or cardiovascular disease
Body habitus	Eating disorders, polycystic ovaries, or Cushing's syndrome
Skin	
Diaphoresis	Fever, withdrawal, NMS
Dry, flushed skin	Anticholinergic toxicity, heat stroke
Pallor	Anemia
Changes in hair, nails, skin	Malnutrition, thyroid or adrenal disease
Jaundice	Liver disease
Characteristic stigmata	Syphilis, cirrhosis, or self-mutilation
Bruises	Physical abuse, ataxia, traumatic brain injury
Eyes	
Mydriasis	Opiate withdrawal, anticholinergic toxicity
Miosis	Opiate intoxication, cholinergic toxicity
Kayser-Fleischer papillary rings	Wilson's disease
Neurological	
Tremors	Delirium, withdrawal syndromes, parkinsonism
Primitive reflexes present (e.g., snout, glabellar, and grasp)	Dementia, frontal lobe dysfunction
Hyperactive deep tendon reflexes	Withdrawal, hyperthyroidism

TABLE 1–3. Selected elements of the physical examination and the significance of findings *(continued)*

ELEMENTS	EXAMPLES OF POSSIBLE DIAGNOSES
Neurological *(continued)*	
Ophthalmoplegia	Wernicke's encephalopathy, brainstem dysfunction, dystonic reaction
Papilledema	Increased intracranial pressure
Hypertonia, rigidity, catatonia, parkinsonism	EPS, NMS
Abnormal movements	Parkinson's disease, Huntington's disease, EPS
Abnormal gait	Normal-pressure hydrocephalus, Parkinson's disease
Loss of position and vibratory sense	Vitamin B_{12} deficiency

Note. EPS=extrapyramidal side effects; NMS=neuroleptic malignant syndrome.

the neurological examination are presented in Table 1–4. Signs and symptoms suggestive of a nonpsychiatric medical cause for psychiatric symptoms are presented in Table 1–5.

Mental status examination (MSE): Key components of the MSE are presented in Table 1–6. A more detailed description of cognitive domains is shown in Table 1–7.

Assessment: Document your impressions and diagnoses, including differential diagnosis and rationale. This will often include an Axis I–V assessment.

Plan: Include recommendations for medications, hospitalization, family involvement, psychotherapy, tests to be ordered to clarify diagnosis, and psychoeducation provided. Also include any consultations, follow-up plans, or referrals to document the transfer of care (American Psychiatric Association 2006).

TABLE 1–4.   Neurological examination

Stance and gait

- Observe walking and turning
- Balance with feet together and eyes closed (Romberg test)

Cranial nerves[a]

- Smell (especially in head trauma) (I)
- Check visual fields by quadrant (II)
- Examine fundus (II)
- Visual pursuit (III, IV, VI) (follow the examiner's finger in horizontal and vertical directions)
- Bulk of temporalis and masseter muscles (V) (opening jaw against force; muscle bulk on tight bite)
- Observe grimace of patient showing teeth (VII)
- Rub finger and thumb an inch from the patient's ears for deafness (VIII)
- Observe palate; ask patient to say "ah" (IX, X)
- Push chin against the examiner's hand and test bulk of sternocleidomastoids (XI)
- Observe tongue for abnormal movements or deviation on protrusion (XII)

Motor system: Test tone, power, and reflexes, and note muscle bulk (test in all four limbs)

- Tone: hold arms out, palms down; observe any wrist drop; rotate leg at knee and note foot movements
- Power: hold arms out, with palms down, and ask patient to "play the piano"; with palms up, watch for any flexion, pronation, or drift; elevate legs from couch and see whether they can be maintained in the air against examiner's pressure; tap floor rapidly with soles of feet
- Reflexes: muscle stretch (biceps, triceps, supinator, knee, ankle); pathological (plantar [Babinski sign])
- Coordination: finger-nose test; rapid alternating movements (tap quickly the back of one hand with the palm of the other)

Sensory testing

- Stroke skin on representative parts of the body, especially the distal extremities

[a]Numerals in parentheses refer to the cranial nerves tested.
Source.   Adapted from Cummings and Trimble 2002.

TABLE 1–5. Signs and symptoms suggesting a nonpsychiatric medical cause for psychiatric symptoms

---

Psychiatric symptoms after age 40 (first onset)

Psychiatric symptoms

    During a major medical illness

    While taking drugs that can cause mental symptoms

History of

    Alcohol or drug abuse

    Physical illness impairing organ function (neurological, endocrine, renal, hepatic, cardiac, pulmonary)

    Taking multiple prescribed or over-the-counter drugs

Family history of

    Degenerative or inheritable brain disease

    Inherited metabolic disease (e.g., diabetes, pernicious anemia, porphyria)

Mental signs including

    Altered level of consciousness

    Fluctuating mental status

    Cognitive impairment

    Episodic, recurrent, or cyclic course

    Visual, tactile, or olfactory hallucinations

Physical signs including

    Signs of organ malfunction that can affect the brain

    Focal neurological deficits

    Diffuse subcortical dysfunction, such as slowed speech/mentation/movement, ataxia, incoordination, tremor, chorea, asterixis, dysarthria

    Cortical dysfunction (e.g., dysphasia, apraxias, agnosias, visuospatial deficits, or defective cortical sensation)

Source.   Adapted from Hales and Yudofsky 2003.

TABLE 1–6.   Components of the mental status examination

General description

    Appearance

    Motor behavior

    Speech

    Attitudes

Emotions

    Mood

    Affective expression

    Appropriateness

Perceptual disturbances

    Hallucinations

    Illusions

    Depersonalization

    Derealization

Thought process

    Stream of thought

    Thought content

    Abstract thinking

    Education and intelligence

    Concentration

Orientation

Memory

    Remote memory

    Recent past memory

    Recent memory

Impulse control

Judgment

Insight

Source.   Adapted from Hales and Yudofsky 2003.

TABLE 1–7.   Detailed assessment of cognitive domains

COGNITIVE DOMAIN	ASSESSMENT
Level of consciousness and arousal	Inspect the patient.
Orientation to place and time	Ask direct questions about both of these.
Registration (recent memory)	Have the patient repeat three words immediately.
Recall (working memory)	Have the patient recall the same three words after performing another task for at least 3 minutes.
Remote memory	Ask about the patient's age, date of birth, milestones, or significant life or historical events (e.g., names of presidents, dates of wars).
Attention and concentration	Subtract serial 7s (adapt to the patient's level of education; subtract serial 3s if needed). Spell "world" backward (this may be difficult for non-English speakers). Test digit span forward and backward. Have the patient recite the months of the year (or the days of the week) in reverse order.
Language	(Adapt the degree of difficulty to the patient's educational level.)
Comprehension	Inspect the patient while he or she answers questions.
	Ask the patient to point to different objects.
	Ask yes-or-no questions.
	Ask the patient to write a phrase (paragraph).
Naming	Show a watch, pen, or less familiar objects, if needed.
Fluency	Assess the patient's speech.
	Have the patient name as many animals as he or she can in 1 minute.

TABLE 1–7. Detailed assessment of cognitive
domains *(continued)*

COGNITIVE DOMAIN	ASSESSMENT
Language *(continued)*	
Articulation	Listen to the patient's speech.
	Have the patient repeat a phrase.
Reading	Have the patient read a sentence (or longer paragraph if needed).
Executive functions	Have the patient follow a three-step command.
Commands	Have the patient draw interlocked pentagons.
Construction tasks	Have the patient draw a clock.
Motor programming tasks	Have the patient perform serial hand sequences.
	Have the patient perform reciprocal programs of raising fingers.
Judgment and reasoning	Listen to the patient's account of his or her history and reason for treatment.
	Assess abstraction (similarities: dog/cat; red/green).
	Ask about the patient's judgment about simple events or problems: "A construction worker fell to the ground from the seventh floor of the building and broke his two legs; he then ran to the nearby hospital to ask for medical help. Do you have any comment on this?"

Source. Reprinted from Smith FA, Querques J, Levenson JL, et al: "Psychiatric Assessment and Consultation," in *Essentials of Psychosomatic Medicine.* Edited by Levenson JL. Washington, DC, American Psychiatric Publishing, 2007, pp 1–12. Used with permission.

TABLE 1–8. Common laboratory tests in psychiatric evaluation

Complete blood cell count

Serum chemistry panel

Thyroid-stimulating hormone (thyrotropin) concentration

Vitamin B_{12} (cyanocobalamin) concentration

Folic acid (folate) concentration

Human chorionic gonadotropin (pregnancy) test (specify serum or urine)

Toxicology (serum, urine)

Serological tests for syphilis (RPR, VDRL)

HIV tests

Urinalysis

Chest X ray

Electrocardiogram

PPD (tuberculosis test for public health reasons in inpatient setting)

Note. HIV=human immunodeficiency virus; PPD=purified protein derivative; RPR=rapid plasma reagent; VDRL=Venereal Disease Research Laboratory.
Source. Reprinted from Smith 2007, pp 1–12. Used with permission.

Additional Tests

Laboratory testing: Table 1–8 lists common laboratory tests used in the psychiatric evaluation of new patients.

Brain imaging: Structural imaging using computed tomography (CT) or magnetic resonance imaging (MRI) has clinical utility in ruling out nonpsychiatric disorders. Brain imaging should be considered when patients present with signs and symptoms listed in Table 1–5. Issues to consider in deciding to order a CT or MRI are shown in Table 1–9.

Positron emission tomography (PET) and single photon emission computed tomography (SPECT) are important research tools. These technologies have been able to clearly demonstrate brain abnormalities in most of the major psychiatric disorders. However, at the time of this writing, there is no clinical utility for the use of either PET or SPECT in clinical psychiatric practice.

TABLE 1–9.   Comparison of computed tomography (CT) with magnetic resonance imaging (MRI)

CT advantages

- It is less expensive than MRI.

- It provides better detection of calcified brain lesions.

- It can be, under some circumstances, more useful when differential diagnosis includes the possibility of some meningeal tumors or pituitary disease.

- It can be used when the imaging subject has a pacemaker.

- It does not raise concern about the potentially dangerous "projectile effect" associated with MRI, in which metal objects (e.g., pens, paper clips, or even oxygen tanks) can be rapidly pulled onto the MRI magnets.

- It can be used in patients with metal in their heads (e.g., surgical clips, metal skull plates, shrapnel); with MRI, this metal can be pulled toward the magnet and can also heat up.

- The CT imaging procedure and device typically induce less anxiety than an MRI.

- The CT procedure and device typically require a shorter period of patient cooperation than the MRI.

- CT can have a uniquely useful role in the evaluation of central nervous system trauma.

MRI advantages

- It provides better visualization of lesions in the posterior fossa, brainstem, and temporal and apical brain areas (i.e., areas closely surrounded by skull bone) (Jaskiw et al. 1987).

- It provides better visualization of demyelinating disease (considered the best method of detecting brain lesions associated with multiple sclerosis).

- It may be superior to CT in detecting brain abnormalities related to seizure foci.

- It is considered better at detecting neoplasms (other than certain meningeal tumors) or vascular malformations (even when angiographically occult).

TABLE 1–9. Comparison of computed tomography (CT) with magnetic resonance imaging (MRI) *(continued)*

- It does not require use of X rays. (However, the long-term biological effects of magnetic fields on patients are unknown.)

When weighing the decision to order a CT scan versus an MRI scan in a psychiatric patient, it is often useful to consult with the neuroradiologist who will be involved in the study.

Note that an MRI brain study might be ordered after an equivocal or unrevealing CT scan study (and when brain pathology is still suspected).

Source. Adapted from Hales and Yudofsky 2003. Data from Garber HJ, Weinberg JB, Buonammo FS, et al: "Use of Magnetic Resonance Imaging in Psychiatry." *American Journal of Psychiatry* 145:154–171, 1988.

Assessment of Risk for Suicide

Virtually all major psychiatric disorders carry an increased risk for suicide. As such, a suicide assessment is essential for all patients regardless of diagnosis in order to help identify and treat risk factors. While no single risk factor can predict suicide, several factors have been identified, and all patients must be considered individually (Simon and Hales 2006).

Suicide Risk Factors for Adults

- Prior suicide attempts
- Suicidal ideation with the intent to act (although denial is not uncommon)
- Severe hopelessness and desperation
- Psychosis
- Family history of suicide
- Negative recent life events (e.g., family problems, unemployment, financial problems)
- Self-injurious behavior (e.g., cutting)
- History of physical or sexual abuse
- Impulsivity
- Guns in the home
- Substance abuse
- Lack of social support

DEMOGRAPHICS

The following demographic groups are at higher risk for suicidal behavior than the general population:

- Males (for completed suicide)
- Females (for attempted suicide)
- Divorced people
- Persons living alone

DIAGNOSES ASSOCIATED WITH SUICIDE RISK

The following diagnoses are associated with a high risk of suicide:

- Major affective disorders (major depression and bipolar disorder)
- Comorbid major depression and generalized anxiety disorder or panic disorder
- Chronic alcohol or substance dependence
- Schizophrenia
- Borderline personality disorder
- Other personality disorders
- Any Axis I comorbidity

In patients with hallucinations regarding suicide, it is important to assess the following factors:

- Content of hallucinations (Are there commands to harm self or others?)
- Are the hallucinations acute or chronic?
- Does the patient hear a familiar voice or an unfamiliar voice? (A familiar voice decreases the ability to resist.)
- Does the patient have the ability to resist commands?

Risk factors for suicide change over the life span. For patients over age 65 years, affective disorders remain a significant risk factor in addition to physical illness, loss of important relationships, and social isolation.

Protective Factors Mitigating Suicide Risk

The following protective factors may mitigate suicide risk:

- Family and social support
- Children at home
- Strong religious beliefs
- Cultural beliefs against suicide

Documentation for Patients at Risk for Suicide

Patient safety is a primary concern of psychiatric care and requires thorough documentation, which should include the following information:

- Suicidal ideation
- Suicidal intent
- Suicide plan
- Acts in preparation (e.g., the purchase of a gun)
- Prior attempts and lethality (e.g., intentional lithium overdose when no one was home and found only by accident and required intensive care unit hospitalization and dialysis [high lethality] vs. six ibuprofen tablets taken in front of boyfriend after a fight [low lethality])
- Treatment interventions (e.g., plan for suicide prevention, identify supports, provide crisis contact information)

Sample Psychiatric Initial Evaluation

ID: Mr. A is a 45-year-old married white male who owns a small trucking company.

Chief complaint: "I have anger problems."

Source of information: Patient, previous record

History of present illness: The patient has a history of "anger problems" and states he was previously diagnosed with major depressive disorder. He now presents as an outpatient for treatment. Since he was a child, Mr. A has struggled with irritability, anger dyscontrol, and impulsivity. He denies being violent with others but admits that he easily loses his temper. He also reports that he has experienced "mood swings" since before he was 12 years old. As he has gotten older he has noted discrete periods lasting weeks to months when he feels "invincible." During these times, he also has significantly increased energy, racing thoughts, and increased impulsivity. For example, he has gotten into arguments with police officers who pulled him over for speeding, has visited prostitutes, and has spent thousands of dollars on music that he could not afford at the time. He states that these behaviors were not within the realm of his usual impulsive behaviors. Immediately following these periods, Mr. A experiences times when he feels depressed for weeks to months. These times are accompanied by symptoms of decreased interest, decreased concentration, increased sleep, psychomotor agitation, and increased guilt. He denies any history of suicidal thoughts or suicidal attempts; however, he sometimes feels that life is not worth living. He states he would not kill himself "because of his kids." He currently feels depressed and irritable but denies any intent to harm himself or others.

The patient denies a history of substance use (other than alcohol in high school) or abuse, generalized worrying, obsessions, or compulsions, panic attacks, hallucinations, or delusions.

Past psychiatric history: Mr. A first saw a psychiatrist when he was 14 years old because "I was getting in trouble in school." He does not recall his exact behavior but states, "I was a kid, I would stay out all night." He participated in therapy for a year but did not take any medications at that time. He did not receive any additional treatment until 1 year ago. At that time he was diagnosed with generalized anxiety disorder and started on sertraline. Over the course of the year, he was also prescribed multiple selective serotonin reuptake inhibitors, all in adequate doses and duration. He has found several of these medications partially helpful, but he has continued to struggle with mood swings and irritability.

The patient denies any history of psychiatric hospitalizations or suicide attempts.

Medication: Escitalopram, 10 mg/day
Dates: 2/1–present
Response: Partial
Side effects: Sexual—delayed ejaculation
Mr. A is not currently taking any nonpsychiatric medications.

Allergies: The patient has no known drug allergies.

Psychiatric review of systems: Positive for affective instability, as noted above. Otherwise negative.

Past medical history: The patient denies any history of traumatic brain injury, seizures, thyroid problems, liver problems, diabetes, and kidney problems. He reports that he has not had a physical examination in the past 5 years.

Family history: The patient's father left the family when the patient was 9 years old, and he and his siblings were raised by his mother after that time. According to the patient, his father also had frequent rage attacks and impulsive behavior. This would cause stress on the family because he would make large amounts of money in the oil industry and then lose it all. This happened multiple times. His father was never treated and is now deceased. No known family history of psychiatric hospitalizations or suicide.

Social and developmental history: The patient grew up in Houston, Texas, the oldest of three children. He reports that life as a child was unstable because of his father's erratic behavior. He was and remains close to his mother and siblings. His first sexual encounter was at age 16 with a girl he dated for several years but did not marry. He had friends during childhood and no apparent developmental delays. He used alcohol during high school and denies other drug use. He is married and has two children, a 12-year-old daughter and a 9-year-old son. He graduated from high school and started college, but when his father died he left college and started a small trucking company. He reports that his spouse is supportive of his treatment and is willing to come to sessions if needed. He reports that his marriage has been strained because of his erratic behavior and involvement with prostitutes. He reports multiple driving violations for speeding. He denies any history of physical, sexual, or emotional abuse.

Substance abuse history: No history of substance abuse.

Physical and neurological examination: (findings not outlined here to save space)

MSE: The patient was casually dressed. His eye contact was good. He was friendly, talkative, and cooperative. No abnormal movements were noted. Psychomotor activity was within normal limits. Speech was spontaneous and clear with normal rate, tone, and volume. Mood was euthymic, and affect was congruent and appropriate. Thought processes were logical and goal directed. Thought content was without suicidal or homicidal ideation. No paranoid delusions were noted. No auditory or visual hallucinations were present. Insight and judgment were intact. Sensorium was clear.

Assessment: Mr. A is a 45-year-old Caucasian male with a history of anger dyscontrol and irritability. He also describes a history of periods of mood elevation when he felt "invincible," had increased energy, behaved more impulsively than usual, and experienced racing thoughts. These periods last weeks to months and are followed by times when the patient feels depressed, with associated symptoms of decreased energy, decreased interests, decreased concentration, increased guilt, and increased sleep that last weeks to months. He currently feels depressed and irritable. He denies suicidal thoughts, but does feel "like escaping" sometimes; he states that he would never purposely harm himself because of the effect it would have on his children. The differential diagnosis includes an affective illness (in particular, bipolar disorder), substance dependence disorder, or psychiatric illness due to a medical condition. These symptoms are most consistent with bipolar disorder. Because the mania resulted in dangerous behavior, he meets criteria for bipolar disorder, type I. From the description of his father's behavior, it sounds as if his father may have also had bipolar disorder.

- Axis I: Bipolar I disorder; rule out mood disorder secondary to general medical condition; rule out substance dependence disorder
- Axis II: Deferred
- Axis III: None
- Axis IV: Marital problems
- Axis V: GAF=70

Plan: The patient and his wife were provided with information about bipolar disorder through discussion and written material. More educational information will be provided at future visits.

- Check thyroid function, liver function, blood urea nitrogen/creatinine levels, electrolytes, HIV status, urine toxicology, rapid plasma reagent, Venereal Disease Research Laboratory (VDRL) results, and complete blood cell count (CBC) with platelets to rule out medical etiology of symptoms and ensure safe use of psychotropic drugs.
- If the lab results are normal, start divalproex sodium (Depakote) 500 mg qhs and increase as tolerated after discussing diagnosis and treatment options.

- Taper and discontinue escitalopram (Lexapro) after Depakote dose is over 1,000 mg, because antidepressant may worsen bipolar disorder in some patients.
- The need for individual and/or couples therapy will be further evaluated.
- Have the patient return to the clinic in 2 weeks.

Admitting Orders

Admitting orders usually address the following issues:

- Where to admit patient (e.g., floor or unit) and name of admitting physician
- Diagnoses, including differentials
- Condition of patient
- Medication allergies
- Diet (e.g., American Diabetes Association diet)
- Patient monitoring parameters
  - Vital signs, weight (how frequent)
  - Restricted to unit or able to leave
  - Presence or absence of suicide precautions

- Consultations (including further medical or neurological evaluations)
- Any additional evaluations (e.g., neuropsychiatric testing, psychological testing)
- Physiological tests (lab work, electrocardiogram, MRI, etc.)
- Medical needs (e.g., diabetic regimen)
- Medications (routine and as-needed [prn] medications, including common over-the-counter drugs such as acetaminophen)
  - Always include a prn order in case the patient becomes agitated. This avoids the delay caused by having the nurses call the physician.

Many facilities have standardized admitting orders, which can help make this process more efficient.

Physical Examination

A physical examination should be completed for all inpatients for the following reasons:

- A medical condition may influence or cause psychiatric symptoms.
- A medical condition may require care.
- A medical condition may influence the choice of treatment.
- The medical evaluation contributes to the assessment of some conditions, such as eating disorders and self-injurious behavior.

Seclusion and Restraint Orders

The use of seclusion and restraint is strictly regulated by federal requirements in addition to the Joint Commission and state requirements. Policies and procedures regarding the use of seclusion and restraint must be adhered to strictly.

Seclusion is the involuntary confinement of a person alone in a room where the person is physically prevented from leaving. Restraint refers to the direct application of physical force to an individual to prevent restriction of movement. Physical force may be human touch or mechanical device; even if mechanical restraints are not used, the patient may still be "restrained" (Simon and Shuman 2007).

Seclusion and restraint are used only when all other measures have failed to prevent harm to self or others or when less restrictive means are ineffective or inappropriate (Simon and Shuman 2007). If your facility has standardized (preprinted) orders for seclusion and restraint, use them—this will help you cover all the requirements. The following points regarding seclusion and restraint should also be observed:

- A face-to-face physician examination must occur within 1 hour of initiation of seclusion or restraint.
  - A member of the nursing staff may initiate an order for seclusion and restraint (as delineated in hospital policy) and should then contact the physician immediately.
  - If you are called about seclusion and restraint, clarify the time the procedure was initiated so that you can arrive within 1 hour.

- After you see the patient, document your visit and describe the patient's mental and physical status and the need for further restrictiveness.
- Your notes should include specific behaviors that demonstrate imminent harm to self or others (e.g., "the patient attempted to hit another patient during lunch").
- Seclusion and restraint must end at the earliest time possible and cannot be written for a certain amount of time (e.g., "seclude for 2 hours" is not acceptable, but "up to 2 hours" is acceptable).
- Seclusion and restraint may not be used for
  - Rude behavior,
  - Staff convenience,
  - Inadequate staffing,
  - Punishment,
  - Behavior modification, or
  - Refusing to do what the staff wants (e.g., take medication, take a shower).

Psychiatric Progress Notes

Inpatient Notes

Inpatient progress notes typically follow the same format as medical notes (the so-called SOAP format):

S Subjective: what the patient says (e.g., "I feel better. I am not hearing voices any more.")

O Objective: what you observe (e.g., "patient appears internally preoccupied but alert and coherent, no evidence of abnormal movements"); includes MSE and vital signs

A Assessment (e.g., "patient still has symptoms but is tolerating treatment well")

P Plan (e.g., "continue antipsychotic")

Outpatient Notes

Outpatient notes typically include the reason(s) for the visit (e.g., medication follow-up or psychotherapy), the duration of the visit in minutes, current medications, response to treatment (including side effects), medication blood levels (if applicable), MSE, assessment, and plan. The following points regarding outpatient notes should also be observed:

- Provide only patient information and opinions that are relevant to diagnosis and treatment. Provide objective data, such as "the patient reports that…." Sharing your thought process for diagnosis and treatment can be helpful to other treaters and those who review the record at a later date.
- Be aware that patients often have access to their records, so avoid terminology that would be harmful to the patient if he or she were to later read the record.
- Notes should be written contemporaneously and should not be altered after the fact. Late notes should be limited and should reflect the time that the note was actually written.

Privacy and Confidentiality

In general, maintain confidentiality unless the patient gives consent to a specific communication. Under specific clinical circumstances, confidentiality may be attenuated to address the safety of the patient and others.

- According to the Health Insurance Portability and Accountability Act (HIPAA; see www.hhs.gov/ocr/hipaa), information from medical records may be released without a specific consent form for purposes of "treatment, payment, and health care operations." Otherwise, the patient must sign an authorization form.
- When releasing information to third-party payers (e.g., for utilization review or preauthorization decision), it may be important to request specific rather than blanket consent from the patient.
- Psychotherapy notes have special protection under HIPAA.
- Release of information about individuals evaluated or treated for substance abuse disorders is governed by state and federal law.

Informed Consent

In addition to meeting requirements of the law, informed consent in psychiatric care allows patients to be partners in their care and can help foster the therapeutic alliance that is essential to longer-term treatment.

In order to provide valid informed consent a patient must

- Have some decision-making capacity;

- Be provided with information about a particular treatment, including the risks, benefits, and prognosis both with and without treatment;
- Be given information on alternatives; and
- Choose voluntarily and not based on coercion or threat.

It is prudent to get consent in writing (a signed form completed by the patient). For some procedures, such as electroconvulsive therapy, written consent is required. When verbal consent is obtained, this should be documented in the progress note.

When obtaining informed consent, provide enough information about the risks that a "reasonable person" in the patient's position would want to know. It is not necessary however, to explain every possible risk. For example, when discussing the use of a medication, you should review the more common side effects and black box warnings, but you do not need to address every possible side effect. Written material about medications and treatments given to the patient can also be helpful but does not replace face-to-face discussion about risks and benefits (Simon and Shuman 2007).

The law requires that certain patient information be disclosed by the treating physician. The following are examples of statutory disclosure requirements:

- Physical evidence or suspicion of child abuse
- Duty to warn endangered third parties or law enforcement agencies
- Commission of a treasonous act
- HIV infection (some states require that the patient's name be reported) (Simon and Shuman 2007)

Hospital Discharge Note

Discharge notes summarize the care and progress of the patient during treatment. Discharge cannot be based solely on denial of insurance benefits. It is important to document the mental status of the patient at the time of discharge or transfer, including documentation about the safety of the patient.

Notes about care after discharge should be as specific as possible. For example, if the patient is transferred to another facility, document details about when, where, and the mode of transportation. In the case of follow-up care, documentation should include dates of appointments if available and instructions given to the patient.

The components of a hospital discharge note are as follows:

- Multiaxial diagnosis
- Hospital course
- Consults
- Case formulation
- Condition at discharge
- Discharge diet/activities
- Discharge medications (including prescriptions written, number dispensed, number of refills)
- Follow-up appointments
- Any pertinent discharge lab results (e.g., lithium levels, CBC)

Suggested Guidelines for Termination of Patient Treatment

1. Thoroughly discuss treatment termination with the patient.
2. Indicate the following in a letter of termination:
   a. Termination discussion (brief)
   b. Reason for termination
   c. Termination date
   d. Availability for emergencies only until date of termination
   e. Willingness to provide names of other appropriate therapists
   f. Willingness to provide medical records to subsequent therapist
   g. Statement of the need for additional treatment, if appropriate
3. Allow the patient reasonable time to find another therapist (length of time depends on availability of other therapists).
4. Provide the patient's records to the new therapist on proper authorization by the patient.
5. If the patient requires further treatment, provide the names of other psychiatrists or refer the patient to a local or state psychiatric society for further assistance.
6. If the need for further treatment is recommended, provide a statement about the potential consequences of not obtaining further treatment.
7. Send the termination letter certified or restricted registered mail, return receipt requested (Simon and Shuman 2007).

References

American Psychiatric Association: Diagnostic and Statistical Manual of Mental Disorders, 4th Edition, Text Revision. Washington, DC, American Psychiatric Association, 2000

American Psychiatric Association: Quick Reference to the American Psychiatric Association: Practice Guidelines for the Treatment of Psychiatric Disorders, Compendium 2006. Arlington, VA, American Psychiatric Association, 2006

Cummings JL, Trimble MR: Concise Guide to Neuropsychiatry and Behavioral Neurology, 2nd Edition. Washington, DC. American Psychiatric Publishing, 2002

Hales RE, Yudofsky SC: The American Psychiatric Publishing Textbook of Clinical Psychiatry, 4th Edition. Washington, DC, American Psychiatric Publishing, 2003

Simon RI, Hales RE: The American Psychiatric Publishing Textbook of Suicide Assessment and Management. Washington, DC, American Psychiatric Publishing, 2006

Simon RI, Shuman DW: Clinical Manual of Psychiatry and Law. Washington, DC, American Psychiatric Publishing, 2007

Smith FA, Querques J, Levenson JL, et al: Psychiatric assessment and consultation, in Essentials of Psychosomatic Medicine. Edited by Levenson JL. Washington, DC, American Psychiatric Publishing, 2007, pp 1–12

2

Psychotic Disorders

Psychosis is a syndrome and can occur in many disorders (e.g., bipolar disorder, depression). Primary psychotic disorders include schizophrenia, schizoaffective disorder, schizophreniform disorder, delusional disorder, and brief psychotic disorder. The lifetime prevalence of psychotic disorders is shown in Table 2–1.

Schizophrenia

Schizophrenia typically begins in adolescence or early adulthood, but can begin in childhood. The male-to-female ratio is equal, but onset in males tends to be earlier. The disorder has a chronic course, with impaired functioning in all areas of life.

Positive symptoms: Beliefs or experiences that healthy people do not typically have, such as delusions, hallucinations, a thought disorder, and bizarre or disorganized behavior. Positive symptoms are most responsive to current pharmacotherapies.

- Delusion: A fixed false belief that is not shared by others of the same culture.

- Hallucination: A perceptual distortion with no external stimulus; auditory hallucinations are the most frequently reported in schizophrenia. Other types of hallucinations suggest a nonpsychiatric etiology, such as olfactory hallucination with seizure disorders (specifically temporal lobe epilepsy) and tactile hallucinations with alcohol withdrawal. Hallucinations should be distinguished from illusions, in which an actual external stimulus is misperceived or misinterpreted.

TABLE 2–1.   Lifetime prevalence of psychotic disorders

Disorder	Lifetime prevalence
All psychotic disorders	3.06
Schizophrenia	0.87
Schizoaffective disorder	0.32
Schizophreniform disorder	0.07
Delusional disorder	0.18
Brief psychotic disorder	0.05
Psychotic disorder NOS	0.45

Note.   NOS=not otherwise specified.
Source.   Data from Perala et al. 2005.

- Thought disorder: Disturbance of thinking that affects language, communication, or thought content, often exhibited as the following:
    - *Loosening of associations:* Unrelated and unconnected ideas; patients shift from one apparently random subject to another.
    - *Word salad:* Incoherent, incomprehensible mixture of words and phrases.
    - *Clanging:* Association of speech directed by the sound of a word rather than by its meaning (e.g., punning and rhyming).
- Bizarre or disorganized behavior

Negative symptoms are those that reflect the loss of functions and emotions that healthy individuals have. Negative symptoms include flat affect (decreased emotional range), poverty of speech (alogia), anhedonia, avolition/apathy, and impairment in attention.

Historical Descriptions of Schizophrenia

Bleuler (1911/1950) described schizophrenia as dementia praecox, differentiating this illness from bipolar disorder on the basis of course of illness. **Bleuler's "4 As" of schizophrenia** are

- Associations
- Affect

- Autism
- Ambivalence

Schneiderian first-rank symptoms are

- Auditory hallucinations
- Thought withdrawal, insertion, and interruption
- Thought broadcasting
- Somatic hallucinations
- Delusional perception
- Feelings or actions experienced as made or influenced by external agents

A mnemonic for the Schneiderian first rank symptoms is ABCD: **A**uditory hallucinations, **B**roadcasting of thought, **C**ontrolled thought (delusions of control), **D**elusional perception (Schneider 1959).

Course of Schizophrenia

A schematic of the prototypical course of schizophrenia is shown in Figure 2–1.

DSM Criteria for Schizophrenia

The DSM-IV-TR (American Psychiatric Association 2000) diagnostic criteria for schizophrenia are shown in Table 2–2, and the subtypes are further described in Table 2–3.

Differential Diagnosis

It is important to rule out psychoses with known medical causes. Psychotic symptoms may result from substance abuse; intoxication; infectious, metabolic, and endocrine disorders; tumors and mass lesions; and temporal lobe epilepsy. The differentiation of schizophrenia from schizoaffective disorder and mood disorder with psychotic features is based on longitudinal course of illness. Table 2–4 summarizes the differential diagnosis of schizophrenia.

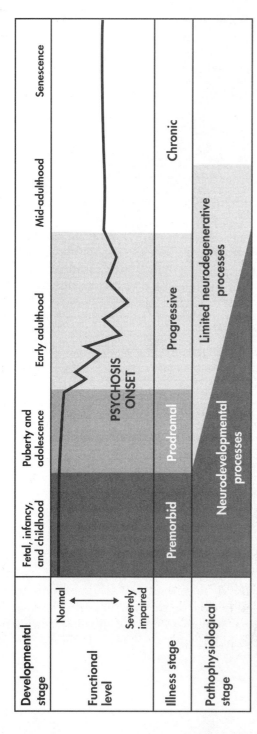

FIGURE 2–1.   Proposed neuroprogressive model of schizophrenia.

The solid line in the upper portion of the figure represents the average functional level over the lifetime of patients with schizophrenia superimposed on the intersection of neurodevelopmental (darkly shaded area to left) and neurodegenerative (lightly shaded area to right) processes. It is hypothesized that the mechanisms that underlie the progressive events are most active around the onset of psychosis and diminish with time.

Source.   Reprinted from Jarskog LF, Gilmore JH: "Neuroprogressive theories," in *The American Psychiatric Publishing Textbook of Schizophrenia.* Edited by Lieberman JA, Stroup TS, Perkins DO. Washington, DC, American Psychiatric Publishing, 2006, pp 137–149. Used with permission.

TABLE 2–2. DSM-IV-TR criteria for schizophrenia

A. *Characteristic symptoms:* Two (or more) of the following, each present for a significant portion of time during a 1-month period (or less if successfully treated):

(1) delusions

(2) hallucinations

(3) disorganized speech (e.g., frequent derailment or incoherence)

(4) grossly disorganized or catatonic behavior

(5) negative symptoms, i.e., affective flattening, alogia, or avolition

Note: Only one criterion A symptom is required if delusions are bizarre or hallucinations consist of a voice keeping up a running commentary on the person's behavior or thoughts, or two or more voices conversing with each other.

B. *Social/occupational dysfunction:* For a significant portion of the time since the onset of the disturbance, one or more major areas of functioning such as work, interpersonal relations, or self-care are markedly below the level achieved prior to the onset (or when the onset is in childhood or adolescence, failure to achieve expected level of interpersonal, academic, or occupational achievement).

C. *Duration:* Continuous signs of the disturbance persist for at least 6 months. This 6-month period must include at least 1 month of symptoms (or less if successfully treated) that meet criterion A (i.e., active-phase symptoms) and may include periods of prodromal or residual symptoms. During these prodromal or residual periods, the signs of the disturbance may be manifested by only negative symptoms or two or more symptoms listed in criterion A present in an attenuated form (e.g., odd beliefs, unusual perceptual experiences).

D. *Schizoaffective and mood disorder exclusion:* Schizoaffective disorder and mood disorder with psychotic features have been ruled out because either (1) no major depressive, manic, or mixed episodes have occurred concurrently with the active-phase symptoms; or (2) if mood episodes have occurred during active-phase symptoms, their total duration has been brief relative to the duration of the active and residual periods.

TABLE 2–2.   DSM-IV-TR criteria for schizophrenia *(continued)*

E. *Substance/general medical condition exclusion:*   The disturbance is not due to the direct physiological effects of a substance (e.g., a drug of abuse, a medication) or a general medical condition.

F. *Relationship to a pervasive developmental disorder:*   If there is a history of autistic disorder or another pervasive developmental disorder, the additional diagnosis of schizophrenia is made only if prominent delusions or hallucinations are also present for at least a month (or less if successfully treated).

Classification of longitudinal course (can be applied only after at least 1 year has elapsed since the initial onset of active-phase symptoms):

Episodic with interepisode residual symptoms (episodes are defined by the reemergence of prominent psychotic symptoms); *also specify if:*   **with prominent negative symptoms**

Episodic with no interepisode residual symptoms

Continuous (prominent psychotic symptoms are present throughout the period of observation); *also specify if:* **with prominent negative symptoms**

Single episode in partial remission; *also specify if:* **with prominent negative symptoms**

Single episode in full remission

Other or unspecified pattern

TABLE 2–3.   DSM-IV-TR subtypes of schizophrenia

Paranoid	Criteria
	• Preoccupation with one or more delusions or frequent auditory hallucinations
	• Relative preservation of cognitive functioning and affect
	• None of the following is prominent: disorganized speech, disorganized or catatonic behavior, flat or inappropriate affect.
	Associated features
	• Often associated with unfocused anger, anxiety, argumentativeness, or violence
	• Stilted, formal quality or extreme intensity of interpersonal interactions
Disorganized	Criteria
	• All of the following are prominent: disorganized speech, disorganized behavior, flat or inappropriate affect.
	• The criteria are not met for catatonic type.
	Associated features
	• Silly and childlike behavior is common; associated with extreme social impairment, poor premorbid functioning and poor long-term functioning.
Catatonic	Criteria
	• The clinical picture is dominated by at least two of the following:
	• Motoric immobility as evidenced by catalepsy or stupor
	• Excessive motor activity (that is apparently purposeless and not influenced by external stimuli)
	• Extreme negativism (an apparently motiveless resistance to all instructions or maintenance of a rigid posture against attempts to be moved) or mutism

---

TABLE 2–3. DSM-IV-TR subtypes of schizophrenia *(continued)*

Catatonic *(continued)*	• Peculiarities of voluntary movement as evidenced by posturing, stereotyped movements, prominent mannerisms or prominent grimacing

Associated features

- Marked psychomotor disturbance is present (stupor or agitation), and unusual motor disturbances may be present.

- Patient may need medical supervision because of malnutrition, exhaustion, hyperpyrexia, or self-injury.

- Sodium amobarbital interview may be helpful diagnostically.

Undifferentiated　Criteria

- Symptoms meeting criterion A are present, but criteria are not met for paranoid, disorganized, or catatonic types.

Associated features

- Probably the most common presentation in clinical practice

Residual　Criteria

- Absence of prominent delusions, hallucinations, disorganized speech, and grossly disorganized or catatonic behavior

- Continuing evidence of the disturbance, as indicated by the presence of negative symptoms or two or more symptoms listed in criterion A for schizophrenia, present in an attenuated form (e.g., odd beliefs, unusual perceptual experiences)

Associated features

- Active-phase symptoms (i.e., psychotic symptoms) are not present, but patient still exhibits emotional blunting, eccentric behavior, illogical thinking, and mild loosening of associations.

Source. Adapted from Hales and Yudofsky 2003.

TABLE 2–4. Differential diagnosis of schizophrenia

Psychiatric illness	General medical illness	Drugs of abuse
Psychotic mood disorders	Temporal lobe epilepsy	Stimulants (e.g., amphetamine, cocaine)
Schizoaffective disorder	Tumor, stroke, brain trauma	Hallucinogens (e.g., phencyclidine)
Brief reactive psychosis	Endocrine/metabolic disorders (e.g., porphyria)	Anticholinergics (e.g., belladonna alkaloids)
Schizophreniform disorder	Vitamin deficiency	Alcohol withdrawal delirium
Delusional disorder	Infectious disorders (e.g., neurosyphilis)	Barbiturate withdrawal delirium
Induced psychotic disorder	Autoimmune disorders (e.g., systemic lupus erythematosus)	Marijuana
Depersonalization disorder	Illnesses caused by toxins (e.g., heavy metal poisoning)	
Obsessive-compulsive disorder	Medications (e.g., steroids)	
Personality disorders		
Factitious disorder		
Malingering		

Source.   Adapted from Hales and Yudofsky 2003.

Evaluation

For a first psychotic break, a workup should include a comprehensive history, family history, mental status examination, physical examination, routine laboratory tests (including rapid plasma reagent), and magnetic resonance imaging or computed tomography.

Treatment

- The long-term outcome for a patient with schizophrenia is better when treatment of the acute episode is initiated rapidly.

- Antipsychotic medications are the foundation of treatment for schizophrenia and other primary psychotic disorders.

- Choice of antipsychotic medication is determined by efficacy, safety, and tolerability profiles.

- Clozapine is generally reserved for patients who have failed to respond to two or more antipsychotic medication trials (Lewis et al. 2006), because of the risk of agranulocytosis (see Chapter 14, "Pharmacotherapy").

- After a patient's first psychotic episode, treatment with the antipsychotic medication should be continued for at least 1 year after a full remission of psychotic symptoms. A trial period without medication may then be considered, except for patients with a history of serious suicide attempts or violent aggressive behavior (Lehman et al. 2004).

- Patients with first-episode psychosis may be more responsive to treatment and require lower doses of antipsychotic medications compared with patients with multiple prior psychotic episodes (McEvoy et al. 1991; Schooler et al. 1997; Zhang-Wong et al. 1999), although the time to response may be longer (Lieberman 1993).

- The American Psychiatric Association Practice Guideline (2004) recommends indefinite maintenance treatment for patients who have had at least two episodes of psychosis within 5 years or who have had multiple previous episodes (Lehman et al. 2004).

- Maintenance therapy should involve the lowest possible doses of antipsychotic drugs, and patients should be monitored closely for symptoms of relapse.

- If the patient is adherent with treatment, oral medications are usually sufficient. However, if the patient's treatment history suggests that the patient may not reliably take daily oral medication, a long-acting depot preparation may be indicated. In most cases, depot preparations of the second-generation ("atypical") antipsychotics are preferred.

- The use of antipsychotics is discussed in detail in Chapter 14, "Pharmacotherapy." However, it is imperative to keep in mind that these medications require monitoring (e.g., blood glucose, body mass index, and abnormal movements). It is essential to educate the patient and family about the risks of developing metabolic syndrome, diabetes, obesity, dyslipidemia, neuroleptic malignant syndrome, extrapyramidal symptoms, and tardive dyskinesia and to document this discussion in the patient's chart.

Treatment Resistance

- A trial of clozapine is recommended for patients who continue to have positive symptoms, frequent relapses, or aggression despite an adequate trial of at least two other antipsychotic medications. Clozapine is also indicated for patients with intolerable side effects due to at least two different antipsychotic medications from different classes (Lewis et al. 2006; McEvoy et al. 2006).

- Electroconvulsive therapy may be considered for patients with catatonia, suicidal ideation or behavior, or persistent severe psychosis or for whom previous treatments, including clozapine, have not been effective (Lehman et al. 2004).

- An additional strategy to use in nonresponsive patients is to add another medication to augment the therapeutic effects of the antipsychotic. Current augmentation strategies include adding lithium, valproate, a benzodiazepine, or lamotrigine. However, use of these augmentation strategies in patients with antipsychotic-resistant schizophrenia should be reserved for patients who cannot take clozapine or who have not fully responded to clozapine (Lehman et al. 2004). If clear benefit is not apparent after 6 weeks of combination therapy, the augmenting agent should be discontinued (Lehman et al. 2004).

- Adjunctive cognitive-behavioral therapy has shown considerable promise when combined with medication in refractory patients (Gould et al. 2001).

- In addition to pharmacotherapy, patients should be referred for vocational and psychosocial rehabilitation. Patients and families should also be referred to the National Alliance on Mental Illness (NAMI) for educational materials and support networks.

Schizophreniform Disorder

Schizophreniform disorder is diagnosed if a patient experiences at least 1 month but less than 6 months of symptoms that are characteristic of schizophrenia. These patients often have an acute onset and resolution of symptoms and usually do not have much functional impairment. Many patients diagnosed with schizophreniform disorder are later diagnosed with schizophrenia or a mood disorder with psychotic features.

The DSM-IV-TR diagnostic criteria for schizophreniform are shown in Table 2–5. The treatment for schizophreniform disorder is the same as for schizophrenia.

Schizoaffective Disorder

Schizoaffective disorder includes key features of both schizophrenia and mood disorders. The key to diagnosis is that a patient with schizoaffective disorder will experience psychotic symptoms in the absence of affective symptoms, whereas patients with mood disorders have psychotic symptoms only while in an acute mood episode (depression, mania, or mixed).

The DSM-IV-TR diagnostic criteria for schizoaffective disorder are shown in Table 2–6.

Differential Diagnosis

As described earlier in this chapter, for schizophrenia, it is important to rule out psychoses with known medical causes. Psychotic symptoms may result from substance abuse; intoxication; infectious, metabolic, and endocrine disorders; tumors and mass lesions; and temporal lobe epilepsy. Schizoaffective disorder is diagnosed instead of a mood disorder if the psychotic features are present for at least 2 weeks outside the active mood episode.

Treatment

Patients with schizoaffective disorder often end up with complex medication regimens in an attempt to target both affective and psychotic symptoms. Treatment options include antipsychotic monotherapy, mood stabilizer monotherapy, antidepressant monotherapy, or combinations. No pharmacological strategy has been found to be superior to another. Acute treatment usually requires an antipsychotic, and maintenance treatment should be guided by the subtype (i.e., mood stabiliz-

TABLE 2–5.   DSM-IV-TR criteria for schizophreniform disorder

A.   Criteria A, D, and E of schizophrenia are met.

B.   An episode of the disorder (including prodromal, active, and residual phases) lasts at least 1 month but less than 6 months. (When the diagnosis must be made without waiting for recovery, it should be qualified as "provisional.")

Specify if:

Without good prognostic features

With good prognostic features: as evidenced by two (or more) of the following:

(1)   onset of prominent psychotic symptoms within 4 weeks of the first noticeable change in usual behavior or functioning

(2)   confusion or perplexity at the height of the psychotic episode

(3)   good premorbid social and occupational functioning

(4)   absence of blunted or flat affect

ers for bipolar subtype and antidepressants for depressive subtype). Longer-term antipsychotics are typically needed.

Delusional Disorder

The core feature of delusional disorder is the presence of a systematized, nonbizarre delusion. The delusion usually fits into a complex scheme that makes sense to the patient, and the patient does not meet other criteria for schizophrenia. A patient with delusion disorder does not typically experience mental deterioration, but the delusion may preoccupy the patient's life. The DSM-IV-TR diagnostic criteria for delusional disorder are shown in Table 2–7.

Capgras syndrome is a delusion that people in the patient's life have been replaced by doubles. This syndrome or "phenomenon" can be seen in many other disorders and diseases, especially dementia, delirium, and brain injury.

Differential Diagnosis

It is important to rule out other causes for delusions, such as substance-induced conditions; dementia; and infectious, metabolic, and endocrine

---

TABLE 2–6.   DSM-IV-TR criteria for schizoaffective disorder

A. An uninterrupted period of illness during which, at some time, there is either a major depressive episode, a manic episode, or a mixed episode concurrent with symptoms that meet criterion A for schizophrenia.

   Note: The major depressive episode must include criterion A1: depressed mood.

B. During the same period of illness, there have been delusions or hallucinations for at least 2 weeks in the absence of prominent mood symptoms.

C. Symptoms that meet criteria for a mood episode are present for a substantial portion of the total duration of the active and residual periods of the illness.

D. The disturbance is not due to the direct physiological effects of a substance (e.g., a drug of abuse, a medication) or a general medical condition.

Specify type:

   Bipolar type: if the disturbance includes a manic or a mixed episode (or a manic or a mixed episode and major depressive episodes)

   Depressive type: if the disturbance only includes major depressive episodes

---

disorders. Abrupt changes in mood, mental state, or personality suggest a nonpsychiatric medical origin. The main focus of diagnosis is to distinguish a delusional disorder from schizophrenia, mood disorders, and anxiety disorders.

Unlike patients with schizophrenia, patients with a delusional disorder do not usually experience hallucinations or disorganized behavior and personality is relatively unchanged. The delusions of mood disorders usually have content that is consistent with the mood disorder, such as delusions of having cancer in the context of major depression, or delusions of being God in mania. If delusions occur only in the context of major depression or mania, the diagnosis is a psychotic mood disorder and not delusional disorder. Patients with obsessive-compulsive disorder may have obsessions that reach delusional proportions, but these patients can usually recognize that their obsessions or compulsions are excessive.

TABLE 2–7.   DSM-IV-TR criteria for delusional disorder

A. Nonbizarre delusions (i.e., involving situations that occur in real life, such as being followed, poisoned, infected, loved at a distance, or deceived by spouse or lover, or having a disease) of at least 1 month's duration.

B. Criterion A for schizophrenia has never been met.
    Note: Tactile and olfactory hallucinations may be present in Delusional Disorder if they are related to the delusional theme.

C. Apart from the impact of the delusion(s) or its ramifications, functioning is not markedly impaired and behavior is not obviously odd or bizarre.

D. If mood episodes have occurred concurrently with delusions, their total duration has been brief relative to the duration of the delusional periods.

E. The disturbance is not due to the direct physiological effects of a substance (e.g., a drug of abuse, a medication) or a general medical condition.

 Specify type (the following types are assigned based on the predominant delusional theme):

    Erotomanic type: delusions that another person, usually of higher status, is in love with the individual

    Grandiose type: delusions of inflated worth, power, knowledge, identity, or special relationship to a deity or famous person

    Jealous type: delusions that the individual's sexual partner is unfaithful

    Persecutory type: delusions that the person (or someone to whom the person is close) is being malevolently treated in some way

    Somatic type: delusions that the person has some physical defect or general medical condition

    Mixed type: delusions characteristic of more than one of the above types but no one theme predominates

    Unspecified type

Treatment

Combined psychosocial and pharamacological treatment appears to be most effective in the treatment of delusional disorder. Antipsychotics are used in the same doses used for schizophrenia. For somatic delusions, addition of a selective serotonin reuptake inhibitor or a serotonin-norepinephrine reuptake inhibitor may be helpful.

Brief Psychotic Disorder

Brief psychotic disorder is characterized by having symptoms for more than 1 day but less than 1 month, with or without a marked stressor. The episode usually has an abrupt onset, and the psychosis is usually bizarre and often accompanied by marked emotional lability. The short duration and return to premorbid functioning are distinguishing features.

The DSM-IV-TR diagnostic criteria for brief psychotic disorder are shown in Table 2–8.

Differential Diagnosis

Like all the psychotic disorders, it is important to carefully rule out medical and substance-induced conditions. Because the onset is acute, carefully consider delirium. If symptoms are present for more than 1 month, the diagnosis changes to schizophreniform disorder. Also consider mood disorders with psychosis if prominent mood symptoms are present.

Treatment

Treatment with an antipsychotic is the primary treatment. Psychosocial treatments should be considered as the patient recovers from the psychotic symptoms.

Shared Psychotic Disorder

Shared psychotic disorder, also known as folie à deux, is a rare condition in which an otherwise psychiatrically healthy person develops delusional ideas that are similar to someone else who has a longer-standing delusion with similar content. Usually the two individuals have close emotional ties.

TABLE 2–8. DSM-IV-TR criteria for brief psychotic disorder

A. Presence of one (or more) of the following symptoms:

(1) delusions

(2) hallucinations

(3) disorganized speech (e.g., frequent derailment or incoherence)

(4) grossly disorganized or catatonic behavior

Note: Do not include a symptom if it is a culturally sanctioned response pattern.

B. Duration of an episode of the disturbance is at least 1 day but less than 1 month, with eventual full return to premorbid level of functioning.

C. The disturbance is not better accounted for by a mood disorder with psychotic features, schizoaffective disorder, or schizophrenia and is not due to the direct physiological effects of a substance (e.g., a drug of abuse, a medication) or a general medical condition.

Specify if:

With marked stressor(s) (brief reactive psychosis): if symptoms occur shortly after and apparently in response to events that, singly or together, would be markedly stressful to almost anyone in similar circumstances in the person's culture

Without marked stressor(s): if psychotic symptoms do *not* occur shortly after, or are not apparently in response to events that, singly or together, would be markedly stressful to almost anyone in similar circumstances in the person's culture

With postpartum onset: if onset within 4 weeks postpartum

References

American Psychiatric Association: Diagnostic and Statistical Manual of Mental Disorders, 4th Edition, Text Revision. Washington, DC, American Psychiatric Association, 2000

Bleuler E: Dementia praecox or the group of schizophrenias (1911). Translated by Zinken J. New York, International Universities Press, 1950

Gould RA, Mueser KT, Bolton E, et al: Cognitive therapy in psychosis in schizophrenia: an effect size analysis. Schizophr Res 48:335–342, 2001

Hales RE, Yudofsky SC: The American Psychiatric Publishing Textbook of Clinical Psychiatry, 4th Edition. Washington, DC, American Psychiatric Publishing, 2003

Lehman AF, Lieberman JA, Dixon LB, et al: Practice guideline for the treatment of patients with schizophrenia, 2nd edition. Am J Psychiatry 161 (2 suppl):1–56, 2004

Lewis, SW, Barnes TR, Davies L, et al: Randomized controlled trials of conventional antipsychotic versus clozapine, in people with schizophrenia responding poorly to, or tolerant of, current drug treatment. Schizophr Bull 32:715–723, 2006

Lieberman JA: Prediction of outcome in first-episode schizophrenia. J Clin Psychiatry 54(suppl):13–17, 1993

McEvoy JP, Hogarty GE, Steingard S: Optimal dose of neuroleptic in acute schizophrenia: a controlled study of the neuroleptic threshold and higher haloperidol dose. Arch Gen Psychiatry 48:739-745, 1991

McEvoy JP, Lieberman JA, Stroup TS, et al: Effectiveness of clozapine versus olanzapine, quetiapine, and risperidone in patients with chronic schizophrenia who did not respond to prior atypical antipsychotic treatment. Am J Psychiatry 163:600–610, 2006

Perala J, Suvisaari J, Saarnia SI, et al: Lifetime prevalence of psychotic and bipolar I disorders in a general population. Arch Gen Psychiatry 64:19–28, 2005

Schneider K: Clinical Psychopathology. New York, Grune & Stratton, 1959

Schooler NR, Keith SJ, Severe JB, et al: Relapse and rehospitalization during maintenance treatment of schizophrenia: the effects of dose reduction and family treatment. Arch Gen Psychiatry 54:453–463, 1997

Zhang-Wong J, Zipursky RB, Beiser M, et al: Optimal haloperidol dosage in first-episode psychosis. Can J Psychiatry 44:164–167, 1999

3

Mood Disorders

Mood disorders are illnesses that significantly impact an individual's outlook on life, confidence, thought processes, interest level, sleep, and appetite. These conditions have a spectrum of severity, but they can be disabling and life threatening. The suicide rate in mood disorders is over 10 times that of the general population.

The first conceptual division in mood disorders is unipolar versus bipolar. Unipolar refers to depression and depressive spectrum disorders. Bipolar disorder, formerly called *manic-depressive disorder* or *manic-depressive illness*, refers to illnesses that include a manic or hypomanic period(s).

The female-to-male ratio is equal for bipolar disorders (1:1), but the ratio is 2:1 female:male for unipolar depression. Table 3–1 shows the lifetime prevalence of mood disorders.

Major Depression

The DSM-IV-TR (American Psychiatric Association 2000) criteria for major depression are shown in Table 3–2. The mnemonic for major depression is **SIG E CAPS,** as in a prescription for energy capsules. Of note, most patients with major depression complain of fatigue.

Sleep. Sleep may be increased (hypersomnia) or decreased. If decreased, the pattern is to wake up too early in the morning and not be able to go back to sleep. This is called early-morning awakening. Difficulty falling asleep is not specific to depression.

TABLE 3–1.   Lifetime prevalence of mood disorders

DISORDER	LIFETIME PREVALENCE
Major depressive disorder[a]	16.6
Dysthymia[a]	2.5
Bipolar disorder, types I and II[a]	3.9
Bipolar I disorder[b]	1.0
Bipolar II disorder[b]	1.1
Any mood disorder[a]	20.8

[a]Data from Kessler et al. 2005.
[b]Data from Merikangas et al. 2007.

Interest.   Depressed mood and/or decreased interest are required for the diagnosis of major depression. The presence of ongoing decreased interest in activities that were previously enjoyable to that person is very helpful in differentiating normal sadness from the illness of major depression.

Guilt.   Guilt is often increased and out of proportion to the circumstances.

Energy.   Energy is typically decreased.

Concentration.   Concentration is typically decreased. To screen for this symptom, ask the patient about reading the newspaper or keeping track of the plot of a book or movie.

Appetite.   Appetite is usually decreased, but it can be increased for some patients.

Psychomotor.   Psychomotor movement and thinking are typically slowed. This is often observable. However, in some cases the patient is agitated ("agitated depression") or may have increased psychomotor activity from anxiety.

Suicidal thoughts.   It is very common for patients with depression to think of death or to think that they are better off dead. At its most extreme, there are thoughts of actual suicide and plans to commit suicide. This is not only a diagnostic issue but obviously a clinical imperative to evaluate and institute protective measures, if necessary (see Chapter 1, "Assessment and Documentation").

TABLE 3–2. DSM-IV-TR criteria for major depressive episode

A. Five (or more) of the following symptoms have been present during the same 2-week period and represent a change from previous functioning; at least one of the symptoms is either (1) depressed mood or (2) loss of interest or pleasure.

Note: Do not include symptoms that are clearly due to a general medical condition, or mood-incongruent delusions or hallucinations.

(1) depressed mood most of the day, nearly every day, as indicated by either subjective report (e.g., feels sad or empty) or observation made by others (e.g., appears tearful). **Note:** In children and adolescents, can be irritable mood.

(2) markedly diminished interest or pleasure in all, or almost all, activities most of the day, nearly every day (as indicated by either subjective account or observation made by others)

(3) significant weight loss when not dieting or weight gain (e.g., a change of more than 5% of body weight in a month), or decrease or increase in appetite nearly every day. **Note:** In children, consider failure to make expected weight gains.

(4) insomnia or hypersomnia nearly every day

(5) psychomotor agitation or retardation nearly every day (observable by others, not merely subjective feelings of restlessness or being slowed down)

(6) fatigue or loss of energy nearly every day

(7) feelings of worthlessness or excessive or inappropriate guilt (which may be delusional) nearly every day (not merely self-reproach or guilt about being sick)

(8) diminished ability to think or concentrate, or indecisiveness, nearly every day (either by subjective account or as observed by others)

(9) recurrent thoughts of death (not just fear of dying), recurrent suicidal ideation without a specific plan, or a suicide attempt or a specific plan for committing suicide

B. The symptoms do not meet criteria for a mixed episode

C. The symptoms cause clinically significant distress or impairment in social, occupational, or other important areas of functioning.

TABLE 3–2.   DSM-IV-TR criteria for major depressive episode *(continued)*

D. The symptoms are not due to the direct physiological effects of a substance (e.g., a drug of abuse, a medication) or a general medical condition (e.g., hypothyroidism).

E. The symptoms are not better accounted for by bereavement, i.e., after the loss of a loved one, the symptoms persist for longer than 2 months or are characterized by marked functional impairment, morbid preoccupation with worthlessness, suicidal ideation, psychotic symptoms, or psychomotor retardation.

Major depressive disorder with atypical features: Depression with mood reactivity (e.g., mood brightens up in response to actual or potential positive events) and two or more of the following features:

- Increased appetite/weight gain
- Hypersomnia
- Leaden paralysis (heavy feeling in arms and legs)
- Long-standing pattern of interpersonal rejection sensitivity

Major depressive disorder with melancholic features: Depression with pervasive anhedonia (loss of pleasure in activities) and lack of reaction to stimuli that ordinarily would be pleasurable, and three or more of the following features:

- Distinct quality of depressed mood (different from the kind of sadness associated with grief)
- Depression that is worse in the morning
- Early-morning awakening
- Psychomotor retardation or agitation
- Anorexia nervosa and weight loss
- Excessive or inappropriate guilt

Major depressive disorder with catatonic features: Depression with at least two of the following features:

- Motoric immobility as evidenced by catalepsy or stupor

- Excessive motor activity (purposeless and not influenced by external stimuli)
- Extreme negativism or mutism
- Peculiarities of voluntary movement as evidenced by posturing, stereotyped movements, prominent mannerisms, or prominent grimacing
- Echolalia or echopraxia

Differential Diagnosis

Many medical conditions can contribute to depression. It is important to rule out underlying medical conditions, as well as substance-induced mood disorder (see Table 3–3).

Treatment of Major Depression

- Although all patients with depression should undergo a thorough medical evaluation, no specific tests are required before initiation of therapy with the newer antidepressants.
- Details of antidepressants use are presented in Chapter 14, "Pharmacotherapy."
- The choice of antidepressant medication is based on the patient's psychiatric symptoms, his or her history of previous treatment response, family members' history of response, medication side-effect profiles, and comorbid disorders. Guidelines for choosing antidepressant medication are presented in Table 3–4.
- The newer antidepressants are better tolerated and safer than tricyclic antidepressants and monoamine oxidase inhibitors (MAOIs) and are first-line agents, with or without combined psychotherapy.
- Clinical response is typically delayed for several weeks.
- An adequate trial of an antidepressant medication is 8–12 weeks (Trivedi et al. 2006).
- Cumulative remission rates are approximately 50% after two consecutive treatments (Rush et al. 2006) and subsequently decrease—hence the importance of aggressive early treatment.

AUGMENTATION AND SWITCHING

If the patient does not reach remission after the initial monotherapy, reasonable strategies include switching to a different monotherapy or aug-

TABLE 3–3. Medical conditions that can cause manic or depressive syndromes (partial list)

Neurological disease	Parkinson's disease, Huntington's disease, traumatic brain injury, stroke, dementias, multiple sclerosis
Metabolic disease	Electrolyte disturbances, renal failure, vitamin deficiencies or excess, acute intermittent porphyria, Wilson's disease, environmental toxins, heavy metals
Gastrointestinal disease	Irritable bowel syndrome, chronic pancreatitis, Crohn's disease, cirrhosis, hepatic encephalopathy
Endocrine disorder	Hypo- and hyperthyroidism, Cushing's disease, Addison's disease, diabetes mellitus, parathyroid dysfunction
Cardiovascular disease	Myocardial infarction, angina, coronary artery bypass surgery, cardiomyopathies
Pulmonary disease	Chronic obstructive pulmonary disease, sleep apnea, reactive airway disease
Malignancy and hematological disease	Pancreatic carcinoma, brain tumors, paraneoplastic effects of lung cancers, anemias
Autoimmune disease	Systematic lupus erythematosus, fibromyalgia, rheumatoid arthritis

Source. Adapted from Hales and Yudofsky 2003.

menting with a second agent. Augmentation strategies include addition of lithium, liothyronine (T_3), or buspirone to a selective serotonin reuptake inhibitor (SSRI) or a serotonin-norepinephrine reuptake inhibitor (SNRI). Combination of two antidepressants with different mechanisms of action is also reasonable. The atypical antipsychotics are also used as augmenting agents, even in nonpsychotic patients.

Electroconvulsive therapy (ECT) and vagus nerve stimulation are options for patients with more treatment-resistant disease (see Chapter 16, "Electroconvulsive Therapy and Device-Based Treatments"). Evidence-based psychotherapy (see Chapter 15, "Psychotherapy and Psychosocial Treatments") is clearly effective and should be offered to all

TABLE 3–4. Guidelines for choosing antidepressant medications

Unipolar depression	Choose on the basis of previous response, side effects, comorbid medical and psychotic disorders, and likelihood of remission.
Bipolar depression	Lithium, lamotrigine, olanzapine-fluoxetine combination, or quetiapine
Depression with psychotic features	Antidepressant+antipsychotic, or ECT; avoid bupropion.
Depression+OCD	SSRI, clomipramine
Depression+panic disorder	SSRI, TCA
Depression+eating disorder	Avoid bupropion.
Depression+seizures	Avoid bupropion and TCAs.
Depression+Parkinson's disease	Bupropion
Depression+sexual dysfunction	Bupropion, mirtazapine
Depression+pain or fibromyalgia	Duloxetine
Depression with melancholic features	TCA[a]
Depression with atypical features	SSRI, MAOI[b]

Note. ECT=electroconvulsive therapy; MAOI=monoamine oxidase inhibitor; OCD=obsessive-compulsive disorder; SSRI=selective serotonin reuptake inhibitor; TCA=tricyclic antidepressant.

[a]Although some data suggest that TCAs are superior for treating melancholic depression, most clinicians choose newer agents because of improved tolerability and safety.

[b]Although MAOIs are highly effective, they are not used as first-line agents because greater risk is associated with their use than with the use of newer agents.

patients as an initial treatment with or without medication and added to the medication treatment for patients with chronic disease and those who do not respond to pharmacotherapy alone.

ANTIDEPRESSANTS AND SUICIDAL BEHAVIOR IN ADOLESCENTS AND YOUNG ADULTS

Patients with depression and other psychiatric disorders are at an increased risk for suicide and suicidal behavior. While long-term pharmacological treatment is associated with a decreased suicide rate (Angst et al. 2002), the acute phases of treatment with antidepressants have been associated with increased risks of suicidal thoughts and behaviors. This is of particular concern in children and adolescents. A pooled analysis conducted by the U.S. Food and Drug Administration (FDA; 2004) of 24 short-term placebo-controlled clinical trials among children and adolescents treated with antidepressants found a risk of suicidal thinking or behavior in 4% of patients treated with antidepressants, compared with 2% of placebo-treated patients. Fortunately, there were no completed suicides in these studies.

At this time, it is not possible to determine if any one medication or class of medications differs with regard to the risk of early treatment-emergent suicidality, so warnings apply to all antidepressant medications. Analyses of FDA data (2007) from adult placebo-controlled trials have shown an increased risk in patients ages 18–24 years, although of a smaller magnitude than in patients under age 18 years. These warnings are not intended to prevent the use of antidepressants, but rather to underscore the need for thoughtful patient education and monitoring. Specifically, the patient should be educated to call the clinician immediately if he or she experiences an increase in suicidal impulses, agitation, or severe restlessness. Family education is also warranted for pediatric patients or those with cognitive impairment.

DEPRESSION WITH PSYCHOTIC FEATURES

ECT is often the acute treatment of choice for depression with psychotic features. If not using ECT, combine antidepressant and antipsychotics. Long-term treatment with antipsychotic medications is generally not warranted, but prophylactic antidepressant medication must be continued as in nonpsychotic depression.

MAINTENANCE TREATMENT OF MAJOR DEPRESSION

- For a first episode of depression, antidepressant therapy should not be discontinued before 4–5 symptom-free months have passed (Prien and Kupfer 1986).
- Antidepressant medication should be continued at the same dose that resulted in remission.
- After one episode of depression, there is a 50% chance that the patient will have a second episode; after three episodes, there is a 90% chance of recurrence (Depression Guideline Panel 1993). Therefore, maintenance treatment is needed for these individuals.
- Indications for maintenance treatment (at least 5 years):
  - Three or more episodes of major depression
  - Two or more episodes and a family history of mood disorder
  - Also consider if there is a rapid recurrence of depressive episodes, an older age at onset, or severe episodes (Keller 2001).
- Some patients may require lifelong antidepressant maintenance treatment.

DISCONTINUATION OF ANTIDEPRESSANTS

When discontinuing an antidepressant medication, it is advisable to taper the dose while monitoring for signs and symptoms of relapse. Abrupt discontinuation is more likely to lead to antidepressant discontinuation symptoms.

- Symptoms of antidepressant discontinuation include nausea, diarrhea, insomnia, malaise, muscle aches, anxiety, irritability, dizziness, vertigo, and vivid dreams. Often, and for unknown reasons, patients who experience this constellation of symptoms have transient "electric shock" sensations. This unique symptom is diagnostically useful and strongly suggests to the clinician that the patient is in fact experiencing withdrawal, because the symptom rarely occurs in other conditions, such as viral infections, or as a side effect of a new medication.
- The symptoms occur most commonly after discontinuation of short-half-life serotonergic drugs (Coupland et al. 1996), such as paroxetine, and venlafaxine.
- The symptoms usually occur within 1–2 days after abrupt discontinuation of a medication and subside within 7–10 days. In some

instances, symptoms may also occur during tapering and dose reduction, and they may persist for up to 3 weeks.

- To treat the discontinuation symptoms, restart the medication and then taper more slowly. Administer one dose of fluoxetine (which has a longer half-life) if discontinuing a medication with a short half-life. Consider using a benzodiazepine for 1 week to help decrease symptoms.

ANTIDEPRESSANT SWITCHING

Often clinicians choose to discontinue the first medication before introducing the second one. In most instances, however, a medication-free period is not critical, if neither medication is an MAOI. Thus, it is possible to start administering the new drug while tapering the dose of the first. This overlapping of medications is sometimes helpful to minimize patient discomfort but must be weighed against the risk of increased side effects and drug interactions (Marangell 2001).

- Switching from one SSRI or SNRI to another can be accomplished by a direct swap of one drug for the next.
- Cross-taper when medications with different receptor effects are used (e.g., an SSRI to bupropion).
- A 2-week washout is required when switching from an MAOI to another antidepressant.
- When switching from another antidepressant to an MAOI, the first medication must be out of the body (i.e., five half-lives).

Dysthymia

Dysthymia is a more chronic but less severe form of depression. The DSM-IV-TR diagnostic criteria for dysthymic disorder are shown in Table 3–5.

Differential Diagnosis

For information on differential diagnosis, see the "Major Depression" section earlier in this chapter. Dysthymia and major depression have similar symptoms but differ with regard to the onset, duration, persistence, and severity. The earlier "Treatment of Major Depression" subsection is also relevant to the treatment of dysthymia.

TABLE 3–5. **DSM-IV-TR criteria for dysthymic disorder**

A. Depressed mood for most of the day, for more days than not, as indicated either by subjective account or observation by others, for at least 2 years. **Note:** In children and adolescents, mood can be irritable and duration must be at least 1 year.

B. Presence, while depressed, of two (or more) of the following:

   (1) poor appetite or overeating

   (2) insomnia or hypersomnia

   (3) low energy or fatigue

   (4) low self-esteem

   (5) poor concentration or difficulty making decisions

   (6) feelings of hopelessness

C. During the 2-year period (1 year for children or adolescents) of the disturbance, the person has never been without the symptoms in criteria A and B for more than 2 months at a time.

D. No major depressiveepisode has been present during the first 2 years of the disturbance (1 year for children and adolescents); i.e., the disturbance is not better accounted for by chronic major depressive disorder, or major depressive disorder, in partial remission.

   Note: There may have been a previous major depressive episode provided there was a full remission (no significant signs or symptoms for 2 months) before development of the dysthymic disorder. In addition, after the initial 2 years (1 year in children or adolescents) of dysthymic disorder, there may be superimposed episodes of major depressive disorder, in which case both diagnoses may be given when the criteria are met for a major depressive episode.

E. There has never been a manic episode, a mixed episode, or a hypomanic episode, and criteria have never been met for cyclothymic disorder.

F. The disturbance does not occur exclusively during the course of a chronic psychotic disorder, such as schizophrenia or delusional disorder.

G. The symptoms are not due to the direct physiological effects of a substance (e.g., a drug of abuse, a medication) or a general medical condition (e.g., hypothyroidism).

TABLE 3–5.   DSM-IV-TR criteria for dysthymic disorder *(continued)*

H. The symptoms cause clinically significant distress or impairment in social, occupational, or other important areas of functioning.

Specify if:

> **Early onset:**   if onset is before age 21 years
>
> **Late onset:**   if onset is age 21 years or older

Specify (for most recent 2 years of dysthymic disorder):

> **With atypical features**

Treatment

See Treatment of Major Depression section above.

Bipolar Disorder

The diagnosis of bipolar disorder is based on longitudinal history, not cross-sectional presentation. If the patient has ever had an episode of mania or hypomania that was not induced by drugs or medication, the diagnosis is in the bipolar spectrum, not the depressive spectrum, *even if* depression symptoms have been more prominent over the recent years (which is common in bipolar disorder). A schematic representation of the subtypes of bipolar spectrum disorders is shown in Figure 3–1.

- Bipolar I disorder is diagnosed if the patient has ever had a manic or mixed episode that was severe enough to impact social and occupational functioning.
- Bipolar II disorder is diagnosed if the patient has only had hypomania.
- The mnemonic for a manic episode is **DIG FAST:**

    Distractibility
    Impulsivity
    Grandiosity
    Flight of ideas/racing thoughts
    Activity (increased goal-directed activity)
    Sleep (decreased need for sleep, as opposed to decreased sleep with fatigue)
    Talkativeness

Bipolar Disorders

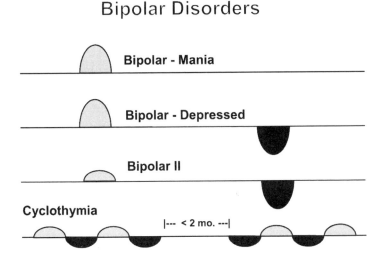

Figure 3–1.   Subtypes of bipolar spectrum disorders.

The DSM-IV-TR criteria for hypomanic, manic, and mixed episodes are shown in Tables 3–6 through 3–8. The DSM-IV-TR diagnostic criteria for bipolar I disorder and bipolar II disorder are shown in Tables 3–9 (summary of criteria) and 3–10 (actual criteria).

Differential Diagnosis

Many substances of abuse and some medications (e.g. stimulants, steroids, L-dopa, antidepressants) can induce manic-like mood disturbances. It is important to rule out underlying medical conditions, as well as substance-induced states (see Table 3–3).

Acute Mania Treatment

- In mild to moderate mania, initiate treatment with a mood stabilizer with acute antimanic properties. These currently include lithium, valproate, carbamazepine, olanzapine, risperidone, aripiprazole, quetiapine, and ziprasidone. If the patient is already taking one of these medications, use the maximal tolerated dose and then combine a second agent, usually either lithium or valproate with an atypical antipsychotic.

TABLE 3–6. DSM-IV-TR criteria for hypomanic episode

A. A distinct period of persistently elevated, expansive, or irritable mood, lasting throughout at least 4 days, that is clearly different from the usual nondepressed mood.

B. During the period of mood disturbance, three (or more) of the following symptoms have persisted (four if the mood is only irritable) and have been present to a significant degree:

   (1) inflated self-esteem or grandiosity

   (2) decreased need for sleep (e.g., feels rested after only 3 hours of sleep)

   (3) more talkative than usual or pressure to keep talking

   (4) flight of ideas or subjective experience that thoughts are racing

   (5) distractibility (i.e., attention too easily drawn to unimportant or irrelevant external stimuli)

   (6) increase in goal-directed activity (either socially, at work or school, or sexually) or psychomotor agitation

   (7) excessive involvement in pleasurable activities that have a high potential for painful consequences (e.g., the person engages in unrestrained buying sprees, sexual indiscretions, or foolish business investments)

C. The episode is associated with an unequivocal change in functioning that is uncharacteristic of the person when not symptomatic.

D. The disturbance in mood and the change in functioning are observable by others.

E. The episode is not severe enough to cause marked impairment in social or occupational functioning, or to necessitate hospitalization, and there are no psychotic features.

F. The symptoms are not due to the direct physiological effects of a substance (e.g., a drug of abuse, a medication, or other treatment) or a general medical condition (e.g., hyperthyroidism).

   Note: Hypomanic-like episodes that are clearly caused by somatic antidepressant treatment (e.g., medication, electroconvulsive therapy, light therapy) should not count toward a diagnosis of bipolar II disorder.

TABLE 3–7.   DSM-IV-TR criteria for manic episode

A.   A distinct period of abnormally and persistently elevated, expansive, or irritable mood, lasting at least 1 week (or any duration if hospitalization is necessary).

B.   During the period of mood disturbance, three (or more) of the following symptoms have persisted (four if the mood is only irritable) and have been present to a significant degree:

 (1)   inflated self-esteem or grandiosity

 (2)   decreased need for sleep (e.g., feels rested after only 3 hours of sleep)

 (3)   more talkative than usual or pressure to keep talking

 (4)   flight of ideas or subjective experience that thoughts are racing

 (5)   distractibility (i.e., attention too easily drawn to unimportant or irrelevant external stimuli)

 (6)   increase in goal-directed activity (either socially, at work or school, or sexually) or psychomotor agitation

 (7)   excessive involvement in pleasurable activities that have a high potential for painful consequences (e.g., engaging in unrestrained buying sprees, sexual indiscretions, or foolish business investments)

C.   The symptoms do not meet criteria for a mixed episode.

D.   The mood disturbance is sufficiently severe to cause marked impairment in occupational functioning or in usual social activities or relationships with others, or to necessitate hospitalization to prevent harm to self or others, or there are psychotic features.

E.   The symptoms are not due to the direct physiological effects of a substance (e.g., a drug of abuse, a medication, or other treatment) or a general medical condition (e.g., hyperthyroidism).

 Note: Manic-like episodes that are clearly caused by somatic antidepressant treatment (e.g., medication, electroconvulsive therapy, light therapy) should not count toward a diagnosis of bipolar I disorder.

TABLE 3–8.   DSM-IV-TR criteria for mixed episode

A. The criteria are met both for a manic episode and for a major depressive episode (except for duration) nearly every day during at least a 1-week period.

B. The mood disturbance is sufficiently severe to cause marked impairment in occupational functioning or in usual social activities or relationships with others, or to necessitate hospitalization to prevent harm to self or others, or there are psychotic features.

C. The symptoms are not due to the direct physiological effects of a substance (e.g., a drug of abuse, a medication, or other treatment) or a general medical condition (e.g., hyperthyroidism).

> **Note:**   Mixed-like episodes that are clearly caused by somatic antidepressant treatment (e.g., medication, electroconvulsive therapy, light therapy) should not count toward a diagnosis of bipolar I disorder.

- In patients who are severely ill or who have manic or mixed states with psychotic features, the American Psychiatric Association (2002) Practice Guideline recommends initial treatment with the combination of lithium or valproate and an atypical antipsychotic.

- The clinical response to antimanic agents may not be apparent for 1–2 weeks; thus, additional medications, such as lorazepam or clonazepam, may be effective adjuncts acutely if certain symptoms, such as severe agitation, warrant immediate control.

- Antidepressants exacerbate mania and should be tapered and discontinued in patients who are in a manic or mixed state.

- ECT is an effective treatment for acute mania and is especially useful for patients who cannot safely wait until medication becomes effective.

- Bipolar disorder typically requires lifelong pharmacotherapy to decrease the risk of future episodes.

- Patient and family education about the illness is essential.

Bipolar Depression Treatment

- The first pharmacological intervention should be to start or optimize treatment with a mood stabilizer rather than to start administering an antidepressant medication.

TABLE 3–9. **Summary of DSM-IV-TR criteria for bipolar I disorder**

A. Presence (or history) of one or more manic or mixed episodes

B. The symptoms cause clinically significant distress or impairment in social, occupational, or other important areas of functioning

C. The mood symptoms are not better accounted for by schizoaffective disorder and are not superimposed on schizophrenia, schizophreniform disorder, delusional disorder, or psychotic disorder not otherwise specified.

Specify current or most recent episode:

Manic: if currently (or most recently) in a manic episode

Mixed: if currently (or most recently) in a mixed episode

Hypomanic: if currently (or most recently) in a hypomanic episode

Depressed: if currently (or most recently) in a major depressive episode

Note. In DSM-IV-TR, diagnostic criteria for bipolar I disorder specify the type of the current or most recent episode (manic, hypomanic, mixed, or depressed).

- Lithium, lamotrigine, the olanzapine-fluoxetine combination, and quetiapine are first-line treatments for bipolar depression. Data are less compelling regarding the use of valproate and carbamazepine for the acute treatment of bipolar depression.

- Lamotrigine can be combined with other mood stabilizers, but it is important to remember that lamotrigine therapy is started at lower doses and dose titration is more gradual when this medication is added to valproate therapy.

- The combination of olanzapine and fluoxetine is particularly useful in patients who are not currently taking other psychiatric medications and who would benefit from a single pill rather than more traditional combined treatments.

- Some patients with bipolar disorder will need antidepressants, but they are not first-line agents because their efficacy beyond mood stabilizers is not clear (Sachs et al. 2007) and they may worsen the course of illness in some patients.

- Tricyclic antidepressants should be avoided when other viable treatment options exist, because they appear most likely to worsen the course of illness.

TABLE 3–10.   DSM-IV-TR criteria for bipolar II disorder

A. Presence (or history) of one or more major depressive episodes.

B. Presence (or history) of at least one hypomanic episode.

C. There has never been a manic episode or a mixed episode.

D. The mood symptoms in criteria A and B are not better accounted for by schizoaffective disorder and are not superimposed on schizophrenia, schizophreniform disorder, delusional disorder, or psychotic disorder not otherwise specified.

E. The symptoms cause clinically significant distress or impairment in social, occupational, or other important areas of functioning.

Specify current or most recent episode:

> **Hypomanic:**   if currently (or most recently) in a hypomanic episode
>
> **Depressed:**   if currently (or most recently) in a major depressive episode

If the full criteria are currently met for a major depressive episode, *specify* its current clinical status and/or features:

> **Mild, moderate, severe without psychotic features/severe with psychotic features**
> **Note:** Fifth-digit codes cannot be used here because the code for bipolar II disorder already uses the fifth digit.
>
> **Chronic**
>
> **With catatonic features**
>
> **With melancholic features**
>
> **With atypical features**
>
> **With postpartum onset**

If the full criteria are not currently met for a hypomanic or major depressive episode, *specify* the clinical status of the bipolar II disorder and/ or features of the most recent major depressive episode (only if it is the most recent type of mood episode):

> **In partial remission, in full remission**
> **Note:** Fifth-digit codes specified cannot be used here because the code for bipolar II disorder already uses the fifth digit.
>
> **Chronic**
>
> **With catatonic features**

TABLE 3–10. DSM-IV-TR criteria for bipolar II disorder *(continued)*
With melancholic features
With atypical features
With postpartum onset
Specify:
Longitudinal course specifiers (with and without interepisode recovery)
With seasonal pattern (applies only to the pattern of major eepressive episodes)
With rapid cycling

- ECT should be considered in severe cases.
- Evidence-based psychosocial treatments that have been developed for bipolar disorder can significantly improve the course of illness when combined with pharmacotherapy.

Maintenance Treatment in Bipolar Disorder

- Patients with bipolar disorder require lifelong prophylaxis with a mood stabilizer, both to prevent new episodes and to decrease the likelihood that the illness will become more severe.
- Ninety percent of bipolar patients relapse after stopping lithium therapy; most do so within 6 months.
- Abruptly stopping lithium, and probably other mood stabilizers, is associated with a substantially higher rate of relapse than is tapering.

Cyclothymia

Cyclothymic disorder is marked by chronic mood changes over a long period of time (at least 2 years). Patients typically experience depressive and hypomanic symptoms during this time, but they never meet full criteria for a major depressive episode or hypomanic episode. See the sections on bipolar differential diagnosis and treatment earlier in this chapter for more information.

The DSM-IV-TR diagnostic criteria for cyclothymic disorder are outlined in Table 3–11.

TABLE 3–11.   DSM-IV-TR criteria for cyclothymic disorder

A. For at least 2 years, the presence of numerous periods with hypomanic symptoms and numerous periods with depressive symptoms that do not meet criteria for a major depressive episode.   **Note:** In children and adolescents, the duration must be at least 1 year.

B. During the above 2-year period (1 year in children and adolescents), the person has not been without the symptoms in criterion A for more than 2 months at a time.

C. No major depressive episode, manic episode, or mixed episode has been present during the first 2 years of the disturbance.

 Note: After the initial 2 years (1 year in children and adolescents) of cyclothymic disorder, there may be superimposed manic or mixed episodes (in which case both bipolar I disorder and cyclothymic disorder may be diagnosed) or major depressive episodes (in which case both bipolar II disorder and cyclothymic disorder may be diagnosed).

D. The symptoms in criterion A are not better accounted for by schizoaffective disorder and are not superimposed on schizophrenia, schizophreniform disorder, delusional disorder, or psychotic disorder not otherwise specified.

E. The symptoms are not due to the direct physiological effects of a substance (e.g., a drug of abuse, a medication) or a general medical condition (e.g., hyperthyroidism).

F. The symptoms cause clinically significant distress or impairment in social, occupational, or other important areas of functioning.

References

American Psychiatric Association: Diagnostic and Statistical Manual of Mental Disorders, 4th Edition, Text Revision. Washington, DC, American Psychiatric Association, 2000

American Psychiatric Association: Practice guideline for the treatment of patients with bipolar disorder (revised). Am J Psychiatry 159 (4 suppl):1–50, 2002

Angst F, Stassen HH, Clayton PJ, et al: Mortality of patients with mood disorders: follow-up over 34–38 years. J Affect Disord 68:167–181, 2002

Coupland NJ, Bell CJ, Potokar JP: Serotonin reuptake inhibitor withdrawal. J Clin Psychopharmacol 16:356–362, 1996

Depression Guideline Panel: Depression in Primary Care, Vol 2: Treatment of Major Depression (Clinical Practice Guideline No 5; AHCPR Publ No 93-

0551). Rockville, MD, U.S. Department of Health and Human Services, Public Health Service, Agency for Health Care Policy and Research, 1993

Hales RE, Yudofsky SC: The American Psychiatric Publishing Textbook of Clinical Psychiatry, 4th Edition. Washington, DC, American Psychiatric Publishing, 2003

Keller MB: Long-term treatment of recurrent and chronic depression. J Clin Psychiatry 62 (suppl 24):3–5, 2001

Kessler RC, Berglund P, Demler O, et al: Lifetime prevalence and age-of-onset distributions of DSM-IV disorders in the National Comorbidity Survey Replication. Arch Gen Psychiatry 62:593–602, 2005

Marangell LB: Switching antidepressants for treatment-resistant major depression. J Clin Psychiatry 62 (suppl 18):12–17, 2001

Merikangas KR, Akiskal HS, Angst J, et al: Lifetime and 12-month prevalence of bipolar spectrum disorder in the National Comorbidity Survey replication. Arch Gen Psychiatry 64:543–552, 2007

Prien RF, Kupfer DJ: Continuation drug therapy for major depression episodes: how long should it be maintained? Am J Psychiatry 143:18–23, 1986

Rush AJ, Trivedi MH, Wisniewski SR, et al: Acute and longer-term outcomes in depressed outpatients requiring one or several treatment steps: a STAR*D report. Am J Psychiatry 163:1905–1917, 2006

Sachs GS, Nirenberg AA, Calabrese JR, et al: Effectiveness of adjunctive antidepressant treatment for bipolar depression. N Engl J Med 356:1711–1722, 2007

Trivedi MH, Rush AJ, Wisniewski SR, et al: Evaluation of outcomes with citalopram for depression using measurement-based care in STAR*D: implications for clinical practice. Am J Psychiatry 163:28–40, 2006

U.S. Food and Drug Administration. Public health advisory: suicidality in children and adolescents being treated with antidepressant medications. October 15, 2004. Available at: http://www.fda.gov/CDER/Drug/antidepressants/SSRIPHA200410.htm. Accessed February 15, 2008.

U.S. Food and Drug Administration. FDA proposes new warnings about suicidal thinking, behavior in young adults who take antidepressant medications. May 2, 2007. Available at http://www.fda.gov/bbs/topics/news/2007/new01624.html. Accessed July 22, 2008.

4

Anxiety Disorders

Anxiety disorders include generalized anxiety disorder (GAD), panic disorder, obsessive-compulsive disorder (OCD), posttraumatic stress disorder (PTSD), acute stress disorder (ASD), specific phobia, and social phobia. The prevalence of some of these anxiety disorders is shown in Table 4–1.

Generalized Anxiety Disorder

GAD is a chronic condition. The essential feature is persistent anxiety for at least 6 months along with multiple physical symptoms, such as muscle tension, restlessness, feeling "keyed up," concentration difficulties, insomnia, irritability, and fatigue. Patients with GAD are usually worried about relatively trivial matters and often anticipate the worst. GAD is highly comorbid with other psychiatric and medical disorders.

DSM-IV-TR (American Psychiatric Association 2000) differentiates GAD from everyday anxiety by specifying that the worry seen in GAD must be clearly excessive, pervasive, difficult to control, and associated with marked distress or impairment. The DSM-IV-TR diagnostic criteria for GAD are shown in Table 4–2.

Differential Diagnosis

Patients with GAD may have peaks in their anxiety and may complain of "anxiety attacks" or "panic attacks." However, careful questioning often reveals that these episodes occur gradually and last for hours to days. In panic disorder, an attack typically peaks within 10 minutes of onset and the physiological symptoms decrease after 20 minutes (Hales and Yudofsky 2003).

TABLE 4–1. Prevalence of anxiety disorders

DISORDER	12-MONTH PREVALENCE	LIFETIME PREVALENCE
Generalized anxiety disorder	3.1	5.7
Panic disorder	2.7	4.7
Obsessive-compulsive disorder	1.0	1.6
Posttraumatic stress disorder	3.5	6.8
Social phobia	6.8	12.1

Source. Data from Kessler et al. 2005a, 2005b.

Asking the patient, "When did you have your first panic attack?" can help in the diagnosis because a panic attack is such a dramatic physical sensation that most patients vividly remember their first panic attack and can often tell you the exact circumstances, such as where they were and the date. With other anxiety disorders, patient's memory and descriptions of panic attacks are often more vague.

It is important to ascertain that the focus of the anxiety and worry is not confined to features of another Axis I disorder; for example, the anxiety or worry is not about

- Being embarrassed in public (as in social phobia),
- Being contaminated (as in OCD),
- Being away from home or close relatives (as in separation anxiety disorder),
- Gaining weight (as in anorexia nervosa),
- Having multiple physical complaints (as in somatization disorder), or
- Having a serious illness (as in hypochondriasis),

and the anxiety and worry do not occur exclusively during PTSD.

Treatment

Selective serotonin reuptake inhibitors (SSRIs) and serotonin norepinephrine reuptake inhibitors (SNRIs) are currently the first-line treatment for GAD (see Table 4–3). SSRIs can be augmented with benzodiazepines, buspirone, and certain antidepressants. See Table 4–4 for a comparison of these medications.

TABLE 4–2.   Medications of choice for specific anxiety disorders

DIAGNOSIS	MEDICATION
Generalized anxiety disorder	SSRIs, SNRIs, buspirone, benzodiazepines
Obsessive-compulsive disorder	Clomipramine, SSRIs
Panic disorder	SSRIs, benzodiazepines
Performance anxiety	Beta-blockers, benzodiazepines
Social phobia	SSRIs, MAOIs, benzodiazepines, buspirone, venlafaxine
Posttraumatic stress disorder	SSRIs, anticonvulsants, adrenergic antagonists

Note.   MAOI=monoamine oxidase inhibitor; SNRI=serotonin norepinephrine reuptake inhibitor; SSRI=selective serotonin reuptake inhibitor; TCA=tricyclic antidepressant.

Benzodiazepines are rapidly effective, but they also carry the risks for abuse and sedation. Tolerance to the sedative effects of benzodiazepines often develops, but tolerance to anxiolytic effects generally does not. All benzodiazepines indicated for the treatment of anxiety are equally efficacious. The choice of a specific agent usually depends on the pharmacokinetics and pharmacodynamics of the drug. Though some patients respond to low doses, mean doses for many patients are typically higher. Benzodiazepines should be avoided in patients with a history of recent and/or significant substance abuse, and all patients should be advised to take the first dose at home in a situation that would not be dangerous in the event of greater-than-expected sedation. The long-term use of benzodiazepines is not recommended for most patients, although some patients do benefit from longer-term use.

Unlike benzodiazepines, buspirone is not associated with significant sedation, motor performance impairment, or abuse problems. However, unlike the rapid onset of action associated with benzodiazepines, the response to buspirone typically occurs after several weeks of treatment. For patients who need rapid relief from debilitating anxiety symptoms, buspirone alone may not be the best choice unless benzodiazepines are also being used. Buspirone does not exhibit cross-tolerance with benzodiazepines and other sedative or hypnotic drugs such as alcohol, barbiturates, and chloral hydrate. Therefore, buspirone does not

TABLE 4–3.   DSM-IV-TR criteria for generalized anxiety disorder

A. Excessive anxiety and worry (apprehensive expectation), occurring more days than not for at least 6 months, about a number of events or activities (such as work or school performance).

B. The person finds it difficult to control the worry.

C. The anxiety and worry are associated with three (or more) of the following six symptoms (with at least some symptoms present for more days than not for the past 6 months). **Note:** Only one item is required in children.

(1) restlessness or feeling keyed up or on edge

(2) being easily fatigued

(3) difficulty concentrating or mind going blank

(4) irritability

(5) muscle tension

(6) sleep disturbance (difficulty falling or staying asleep, or restless unsatisfying sleep)

D. The focus of the anxiety and worry is not confined to features of an Axis I disorder, e.g., the anxiety or worry is not about having a panic attack (as in panic disorder), being embarrassed in public (as in social phobia), being contaminated (as in obsessive-compulsive disorder), being away from home or close relatives (as in separation anxiety disorder), gaining weight (as in anorexia nervosa), having multiple physical complaints (as in somatization disorder), or having a serious illness (as in hypochondriasis), and the anxiety and worry do not occur exclusively during posttraumatic stress disorder.

E. The anxiety, worry, or physical symptoms cause clinically significant distress or impairment in social, occupational, or other important areas of functioning.

F. The disturbance is not due to the direct physiological effects of a substance (e.g., a drug of abuse, a medication) or a general medical condition (e.g., hyperthyroidism) and does not occur exclusively during a mood disorder, a psychotic disorder, or a pervasive developmental disorder.

TABLE 4–4. Comparison of benzodiazepines, buspirone, and antidepressants for the treatment of anxiety

CHARACTERISTIC	BENZODIAZEPINES	BUSPIRONE	ANTIDEPRESSANTS[a]
Immediate effect	Yes	No	No
Time to full therapeutic action	Days	Weeks to months	Weeks
Sedation	Yes	No	Unlikely
Risk of dependence	Yes	No	No
Impairs cognitive and motor performance	Yes	No	No
Suppresses sedative withdrawal symptoms	Yes	No	No
Once-daily dosing	No	No	Yes
Treats comorbid depression	No	No	Yes
Common side effects	Sedation, memory impairment, risk of falls and delirium in elderly/medically ill	Nausea, headache, nervousness, insomnia, dizziness, light-headedness, restlessness	Nausea, loose bowel movements, headache, anxiety, insomnia, sexual dysfunction, increased sweating

[a]See text for details.

suppress benzodiazepine withdrawal symptoms. In anxious patients who are being treated with a benzodiazepine and who require a switch to buspirone, the benzodiazepine must be tapered gradually to avoid withdrawal symptoms.

GAD also responds to antidepressant treatment. As with buspirone, response to treatment with antidepressants typically occurs after several weeks of treatment, and maximal response may take months. Venlafaxine, escitalopram, paroxetine, and duloxetine have received U.S. Food and Drug Administration (FDA) approval for this indication, although it is likely that the other SSRIs are effective as well.

The duration of pharmacotherapy for GAD is controversial. Psychotherapy is recommended for most patients with this disorder, and it may facilitate the tapering of doses of medication. However, generalized anxiety is often a chronic condition, and some patients require long-term pharmacotherapy. As in other anxiety disorders, the need for ongoing treatment should be reassessed every 6–12 months.

Panic Disorder

Panic disorder is characterized by recurrent unexpected panic attacks that are discrete and followed by a month of persistent anticipatory anxiety or behavioral change. The diagnostic criteria for a panic attack are outlined in Table 4–5.

While a first panic attack may be precipitated by a significant life stressor, panic attacks often occur out of the blue. It is not unusual for patients to go to the emergency room fearing that they are having a heart attack. Not surprisingly, most patients develop some anticipatory anxiety and phobic avoidance associated with the circumstances of the first panic attack.

The fears and avoidance behavior associated with agoraphobia typically revolve around three main themes: fear of leaving home, fear of being alone, and fear of being away from home in situations where one can feel trapped, embarrassed, or helpless. At its worst, patients may become completely housebound. The diagnosis of panic disorder is specified as with or without agoraphobia (see Table 4–6).

The DSM-IV-TR diagnostic criteria for panic disorder without agoraphobia are shown in Table 4–7, and the criteria for panic disorder with agoraphobia are shown in Table 4–8.

TABLE 4–5. DSM-IV-TR criteria for panic attack

Note: A panic attack is not a codable disorder. Code the specific diagnosis in which the panic attack occurs (e.g., 300.21 panic disorder with agoraphobia).

A discrete period of intense fear or discomfort, in which four (or more) of the following symptoms developed abruptly and reached a peak within 10 minutes:

   (1) palpitations, pounding heart, or accelerated heart rate

   (2) sweating

   (3) trembling or shaking

   (4) sensations of shortness of breath or smothering

   (5) feeling of choking

   (6) chest pain or discomfort

   (7) nausea or abdominal distress

   (8) feeling dizzy, unsteady, lightheaded, or faint

   (9) derealization (feelings of unreality) or depersonalization (being detached from oneself)

 (10) fear of losing control or going crazy

 (11) fear of dying

 (12) paresthesias (numbness or tingling sensations)

 (13) chills or hot flushes

Differential Diagnosis

Panic attacks can occur with other anxiety disorders (specific phobia, social phobia, PTSD), but are typically situationally bound or cued (i.e., panic attacks in panic disorder occur out of the blue and are not limited to phobic situations or reminders of a traumatic event). Medical conditions that mimic panic attacks include cardiac, respiratory, vestibular, and gastrointestinal diseases, but it is important to keep in mind that patients with panic disorder often first present to an emergency room or primary care for a cardiac evaluation. Table 4–9 presents the differential diagnosis of panic disorder.

TABLE 4–6.   DSM-IV-TR criteria for agoraphobia

Note: Agoraphobia is not a codable disorder. Code the specific disorder in which the agoraphobia occurs (e.g., 300.21 panic disorder with agoraphobia or 300.22 agoraphobia without history of panic disorder.

A.   Anxiety about being in places or situations from which escape might be difficult (or embarrassing) or in which help may not be available in the event of having an unexpected or situationally predisposed panic attack or panic-like symptoms. Agoraphobic fears typically involve characteristic clusters of situations that include being outside the home alone; being in a crowd or standing in a line; being on a bridge; and traveling in a bus, train, or automobile.

   Note: Consider the diagnosis of specific phobia if the avoidance is limited to one or only a few specific situations, or social phobia if the avoidance is limited to social situations.

B.   The situations are avoided (e.g., travel is restricted) or else are endured with marked distress or with anxiety about having a panic attack or panic-like symptoms, or require the presence of a companion.

C.   The anxiety or phobic avoidance is not better accounted for by another mental disorder, such as social phobia (e.g., avoidance limited to social situations because of fear of embarrassment), specific phobia (e.g., avoidance limited to a single situation like elevators), obsessive-compulsive disorder (e.g., avoidance of dirt in someone with an obsession about contamination), posttraumatic stress disorder (e.g., avoidance of stimuli associated with a severe stressor), or separation anxiety disorder (e.g., avoidance of leaving home or relatives).

Treatment

Combined psychosocial and pharamacological treatment appears to be most effective for the treatment of panic disorder. The SSRIs are considered first-line treatment. Doses of antidepressants may be started at half the usual recommended dose for depression because patients with panic disorder may be more sensitive to side effects and there is a potential for an initial increase in anxiety side effects. Doses should then be titrated to full therapeutic dose as tolerated by the patient. In combination with other treatment modalities, benzodiazepines may be useful for early symptom control. Weekly cognitive-behavioral therapy, as well as supportive and family therapy, may be beneficial. Benzodiaz-

---

TABLE 4–7. DSM-IV-TR criteria for panic disorder without agoraphobia

---

A. Both (1) and (2):

   (1) recurrent unexpected panic attacks

   (2) at least one of the attacks has been followed by 1 month (or more) of one (or more) of the following:

   (a) persistent concern about having additional attacks

   (b) worry about the implications of the attack or its consequences (e.g., losing control, having a heart attack, "going crazy")

   (c) a significant change in behavior related to the attacks

B. Absence of agoraphobia.

C. The panic attacks are not due to the direct physiological effects of a substance (e.g., a drug of abuse, a medication) or a general medical condition (e.g., hyperthyroidism).

D. The panic attacks are not better accounted for by another mental disorder, such as social phobia (e.g., occurring on exposure to feared social situations), specific phobia (e.g., on exposure to a specific phobic situation), obsessive-compulsive disorder (e.g., on exposure to dirt in someone with an obsession about contamination), posttraumatic stress disorder (e.g., in response to stimuli associated with a severe stressor), or separation anxiety disorder (e.g., in response to being away from home or close relatives).

---

epines, tricyclic antidepressants (TCAs), monoamine oxidase inhibitors (MAOIs), and SSRIs are all effective in the treatment of panic disorder. Among the benzodiazepines, the high-potency agents are preferred because they are well tolerated at the higher doses often required to treat panic disorder. The benzodiazepine may provide the patient with immediate anxiety relief until the antidepressant becomes effective. When panic symptoms have been absent for several weeks, the benzodiazepine dose should then be slowly tapered if possible.

The duration of pharmacotherapy for patients with panic disorder is unknown. The clinician should consider attempting a gradual medication discontinuation every 6–12 months if the patient has been relatively symptom-free. However, many patients may require longer-term pharmacotherapy.

TABLE 4–8.   DSM-IV-TR criteria for panic disorder with agoraphobia

---

A. Both (1) and (2):

  (1) recurrent unexpected panic attacks

  (2) at least one of the attacks has been followed by 1 month (or more) of one (or more) of the following:

    (a) persistent concern about having additional attacks

    (b) worry about the implications of the attack or its consequences (e.g., losing control, having a heart attack, "going crazy")

    (c) a significant change in behavior related to the attacks

B. The presence of agoraphobia.

C. The panic attacks are not due to the direct physiological effects of a substance (e.g., a drug of abuse, a medication) or a general medical condition (e.g., hyperthyroidism).

D. The panic attacks are not better accounted for by another mental disorder, such as social phobia (e.g., occurring on exposure to feared social situations), specific phobia (e.g., on exposure to a specific phobic situation), obsessive-compulsive disorder (e.g., on exposure to dirt in someone with an obsession about contamination), posttraumatic stress disorder (e.g., in response to stimuli associated with a severe stressor), or separation anxiety disorder (e.g., in response to being away from home or close relatives).

Obsessive-Compulsive Disorder

OCD usually begins in adolescence or early adulthood and presents in many different forms. An obsession is an intrusive, unwanted mental event, which usually evokes anxiety or distress. Obsessions can be thoughts, images, ideas, sounds, ruminations, convictions, fears, or impulses. They usually have an aggressive, sexual, religious, "disgusting," or nonsensical content. A compulsion is a behavior that reduces distress and is carried out in a pressured or compulsive manner. Washing and checking behaviors are the two most common types of compulsions. Mental compulsions are also common and often go unrecognized if the clinician only asks about behaviors. An example of a mental compul-

---

TABLE 4–9. Differential diagnosis of panic disorder

Anxious depression

Somatization disorder with paniclike physical complaints

Social phobia with socially cued panic attacks

Generalized anxiety disorder with severe symptoms or during peak periods

Posttraumatic stress disorder with intense physiological response to reminders of the trauma

Depersonalization disorder

Personality disorder with anxiety symptoms

Hyperthyroidism

Hypothyroidism

Mitral valve prolapse

Pheochromocytoma

Vestibular disorders

Panic attack associated with substance use or withdrawal (cocaine use, alcohol withdrawal)

Source. Adapted from Hales and Yudofsky 2003.

sion is the need to count to a certain number before walking through a door. The DSM-IV-TR diagnostic criteria for OCD are shown in Table 4–10.

Differential Diagnosis

The terms "obsession" and "compulsion" are often used to refer to behaviors that are not true OCD. Excessive activities, such as eating, gambling, and sexual activity, that are typically experienced as pleasurable and ego-syntonic may not be true compulsions. Similarly, negative thought patterns associated with depression (obsessive brooding, ruminations, or preoccupations) can be distinguished from true obsessions because they are not as senseless or intrusive and the patient often sees them as meaningful. Sometimes it is difficult to distinguish between an obsession and a delusion. Typically, an obsession is ego-dystonic and the patient realizes the thoughts are not "real," whereas a delusion is regarded as true by the patient. Table 4–11 presents the differential diagnosis of OCD.

TABLE 4–10.   DSM-IV-TR criteria for obsessive-compulsive
disorder

A.   Either obsessions or compulsions:

Obsessions as defined by (1), (2), (3), and (4):

(1)   recurrent and persistent thoughts, impulses, or images that are experienced, at some time during the disturbance, as intrusive and inappropriate and that cause marked anxiety or distress

(2)   the thoughts, impulses, or images are not simply excessive worries about real-life problems

(3)   the person attempts to ignore or suppress such thoughts, impulses, or images, or to neutralize them with some other thought or action

(4)   the person recognizes that the obsessional thoughts, impulses, or images are a product of his or her own mind (not imposed from without as in thought insertion)

Compulsions as defined by (1) and (2):

(1)   repetitive behaviors (e.g., hand washing, ordering, checking) or mental acts (e.g., praying, counting, repeating words silently) that the person feels driven to perform in response to an obsession, or according to rules that must be applied rigidly

(2)   the behaviors or mental acts are aimed at preventing or reducing distress or preventing some dreaded event or situation; however, these behaviors or mental acts either are not connected in a realistic way with what they are designed to neutralize or prevent or are clearly excessive

B.   At some point during the course of the disorder, the person has recognized that the obsessions or compulsions are excessive or unreasonable.   **Note:** This does not apply to children.

C.   The obsessions or compulsions cause marked distress, are time consuming (take more than 1 hour a day), or significantly interfere with the person's normal routine, occupational (or academic) functioning, or usual social activities or relationships.

TABLE 4–10.	**DSM-IV-TR criteria for obsessive-compulsive disorder *(continued)***

D. If another Axis I disorder is present, the content of the obsessions or compulsions is not restricted to it (e.g., preoccupation with food in the presence of an eating disorder; hair pulling in the presence of trichotillomania; concern with appearance in the presence of body dysmorphic disorder; preoccupation with drugs in the presence of a substance use disorder; preoccupation with having a serious illness in the presence of hypochondriasis; preoccupation with sexual urges or fantasies in the presence of a paraphilia; or guilty ruminations in the presence of major depressive disorder).

E. The disturbance is not due to the direct physiological effects of a substance (e.g., a drug of abuse, a medication) or a general medical condition.

Specify if:

> **With poor insight:**   if, for most of the time during the current episode, the person does not recognize that the obsessions and compulsions are excessive or unreasonable

Treatment

Currently, clomipramine and SSRIs provide the foundation of pharmacological treatment of OCD. However, it is important to note that many patients with OCD experience a 60% or less improvement in symptoms (Jenike 1990). Additionally, medication responses may not be apparent until treatment has been given for 10 weeks, and some patients may require doses of SSRIs that are higher than those typically used for the treatment of major depression. Cognitive-behavioral therapy should be combined with pharmacological approaches.

The typical dosage range for clomipramine in the treatment of patients with OCD is between 150 and 200 mg/day. Before initiating clomipramine treatment, the clinician must heed all the precautions and dosing guidelines associated with the use of any TCA (see Chapter 14, "Pharmacotherapy"). Additionally, clinicians should monitor patients for the emergence of anticholinergic, antihistaminic, and α_2-adrenergic side effects.

The SSRIs paroxetine, fluoxetine, fluvoxamine, and sertraline have been approved by the FDA for the treatment of OCD. As noted above, SSRI dosages may be higher for some patients being treated for OCD

TABLE 4–11. Differential diagnosis of obsessive-compulsive disorder (OCD)

Eating disorder with obsessions surrounding food and weight

Body dysmorphic disorder with obsessions about body appearance other than weight

Hypochondriasis with obsessions related to feared illness

Obsessive ruminations of depression (typically mood congruent)

Severe obsessive-compulsive personality disorder

Paranoid psychosis (e.g., delusions of poisoning rather than fears of contamination)

Social phobia (if social settings are avoided because they exacerbate OCD)

Impulse-control disorders (repetitive behaviors associated with pleasure or gratification, such as compulsive gambling, compulsive spending, or compulsive sexual behavior)

Source. Adapted from Hales and Yudofsky 2003.

compared with dosages typically used for the treatment of major depression. For fluoxetine, the recommended dosage range for the treatment of OCD is 20–60 mg/day, though some clinicians target a daily dose of up to 80 mg. Therapeutic dosages of fluvoxamine range from 100 to 300 mg/day in divided doses. The recommended dosage range for paroxetine in the treatment of OCD is 40–60 mg/day. The recommended dosage range of sertraline for the treatment of OCD is 50–200 mg/day.

The exact duration of pharmacotherapy for OCD has not been established. OCD is often a lifelong disorder with a waxing and waning course, for which many patients require prolonged pharmacotherapy.

Posttraumatic Stress Disorder

PTSD refers to a cluster of symptoms that typically develop following a traumatic event and often include reexperiencing of the trauma, avoidance and numbing, and increased autonomic arousal. The trauma is often reexperienced in recurrent painful and intrusive recollections, flashbacks, nightmares, or intense emotional and physiological reactions to reminders of the trauma. The patient tries to avoid thoughts or feelings associated with the event and anything that might arouse recollection of it. There may be amnesia for an important aspect of the trauma. In addition, patients typically experience a psychic numbing and become disinterested and detached from others and their environment. Dissociative states may also occur. Excessive autonomic arousal may present as irritability, exaggerated startle response, poor concentration, hypervigilance, and insomnia.

Approximately 50%–90% of individuals with PTSD have a comorbid psychiatric disorder. Most individuals who are exposed to traumatic events do not develop this disorder. Individual vulnerability and coping style may affect the severity and occurrence of PTSD. The DSM-IV-TR diagnostic criteria for PTSD are shown in Table 4–12.

Differential Diagnosis

Diagnosing PTSD is usually not difficult if there is a clear history of exposure to a traumatic event followed by symptoms of intense anxiety lasting at least 1 month, numbing of responsiveness, and avoidance or reexperiencing of the traumatic event. However, it is important to clearly assess the onset of symptoms as subsequent to the trauma.

There is a high rate of comorbidity with PTSD, which often leads to additional diagnosis of panic disorder, depression, or GAD (see Table 4–13). Symptoms such as irritability, sleep disturbance, fatigue, anhedonia, and pessimistic outlook can occur in both PTSD and mood disorders. Major depression frequently occurs with PTSD and should be treated aggressively because this comorbidity carries an increased risk of suicide. Organic mental disorders should also be ruled out, such as organic personality syndrome, delirium, and amnesic syndrome.

Treatment

SSRIs are recommended as first-line treatment for PTSD and have been associated with relief of the core PTSD symptoms of reexperiencing, avoidance/numbing, and hyperarousal. TCAs and MAOIs may also be useful, but they are not considered first-line treatment. Multiple anticonvulsants (valproic acid, carbamazepine, lamotrigine) have been shown to be of benefit in the treatment of PTSD, but data thus far are predominantly from open trials. Anticonvulsants are typically used in combination with antidepressants, and may help with the residual affective lability and impulsivity that is often seen in PTSD. Adrenergic antagonists are also used as adjunctive treatments based on data from open trials. Agents studied include propranolol, clonidine, and guanfacine. Prazosin may be helpful in the treatment of nightmares associated with PTSD (Raskind et al. 2007). Cognitive-behavioral therapy has been

---

TABLE 4–12.   DSM-IV-TR criteria for posttraumatic stress
disorder

A. The person has been exposed to a traumatic event in which both of
the following were present:

   (1) the person experienced, witnessed, or was confronted with an
event or events that involved actual or threatened death or
serious injury, or a threat to the physical integrity of self or others

   (2) the person's response involved intense fear, helplessness, or
horror. **Note:** In children, this may be expressed instead by
disorganized or agitated behavior

B. The traumatic event is persistently reexperienced in one (or more) of
the following ways:

   (1) recurrent and intrusive distressing recollections of the event,
including images, thoughts, or perceptions. **Note:** In young
children, repetitive play may occur in which themes or aspects of
the trauma are expressed.

   (2) recurrent distressing dreams of the event. **Note:** In children, there
may be frightening dreams without recognizable content.

   (3) acting or feeling as if the traumatic event were recurring (includes
a sense of reliving the experience, illusions, hallucinations, and
dissociative flashback episodes, including those that occur on
awakening or when intoxicated). **Note:** In young children,
trauma-specific reenactment may occur.

   (4) intense psychological distress at exposure to internal or external
cues that symbolize or resemble an aspect of the traumatic event

   (5) physiological reactivity on exposure to internal or external cues
that symbolize or resemble an aspect of the traumatic event

C. Persistent avoidance of stimuli associated with the trauma and
numbing of general responsiveness (not present before the trauma),
as indicated by three (or more) of the following:

   (1) efforts to avoid thoughts, feelings, or conversations associated
with the trauma

   (2) efforts to avoid activities, places, or people that arouse
recollections of the trauma

   (3) inability to recall an important aspect of the trauma

TABLE 4–12. DSM-IV-TR criteria for posttraumatic stress disorder *(continued)*

---

  (4) markedly diminished interest or participation in significant activities

  (5) feeling of detachment or estrangement from others

  (6) restricted range of affect (e.g., unable to have loving feelings)

  (7) sense of a foreshortened future (e.g., does not expect to have a career, marriage, children, or a normal life span)

D. Persistent symptoms of increased arousal (not present before the trauma), as indicated by two (or more) of the following:

  (1) difficulty falling or staying asleep

  (2) irritability or outbursts of anger

  (3) difficulty concentrating

  (4) hypervigilance

  (5) exaggerated startle response

E. Duration of the disturbance (symptoms in criteria B, C, and D) is more than 1 month.

F. The disturbance causes clinically significant distress or impairment in social, occupational, or other important areas of functioning.

  Specify if:

  Acute: if duration of symptoms is less than 3 months

  Chronic: if duration of symptoms is 3 months or more

  Specify if:

  With delayed onset: if onset of symptoms is at least 6 months after the stressor

---

demonstrated to be effective in treating core PTSD symptoms, and often includes some degree of exposure to the feared situations and anxiety management techniques.

Acute Stress Disorder

ASD develops after exposure to a traumatic event and is similar to PTSD in its symptomatology, but it is time limited (lasting up to 1 month after the event). Dissociative symptoms are prominent in ASD and are re-

---

TABLE 4–13.   Differential diagnosis of posttraumatic stress
disorder

Depression after trauma (numbing and avoidance may be present, but not
hyperarousal or intrusive symptoms)

Panic disorder (if panic attacks are not limited to reminders or triggers of
the trauma)

Generalized anxiety disorder (may have symptoms similar to hyperarousal)

Agoraphobia (if avoidance is not directly trauma related)

Specific phobia (if avoidance is not directly trauma related)

Adjustment disorder (usually has less severe stressor and different
symptoms)

Acute stress disorder (if less than 1 month has elapsed since trauma)

Dissociative disorders (if prominent dissociative symptoms are present)

Factitious disorders or malingering (especially if secondary gain is
apparent)

Source.   Adapted from Hales and Yudofsky 2003.

quired for the diagnosis. Many people with ASD develop PTSD, and it
has been argued that these are not two discrete disorders, but they are
currently separate diagnoses in DSM-IV-TR. Most individuals who are
exposed to major stressors do not develop this disorder. Individual vulnerability and coping style may affect the severity and occurrence of
ASD. The DSM-IV-TR diagnostic criteria for ASD are shown in Table 4–14.

Differential Diagnosis

Adjustment disorder involves a short-term anxiety reaction to a life
stressor, but the stressor (e.g., loss of a job, a relationship breakup) is
usually less traumatic than in ASD. ASD should not be diagnosed if the
symptoms are simply an exacerbation of existing symptoms of another
psychiatric disorder (with the exception of personality disorders).

Treatment

There are very few studies of pharmacological intervention for ASD.
SSRIs may be useful in the treatment of ASD, given their efficacy in the
treatment of PTSD. Benzodiazepines may be useful in reducing anxiety

---

TABLE 4–14. **DSM-IV-TR criteria for acute stress disorder**

A. The person has been exposed to a traumatic event in which both of the following were present:

    (1) the person experienced, witnessed, or was confronted with an event or events that involved actual or threatened death or serious injury, or a threat to the physical integrity of self or others

    (2) the person's response involved intense fear, helplessness, or horror

B. Either while experiencing or after experiencing the distressing event, the individual has three (or more) of the following dissociative symptoms:

    (1) a subjective sense of numbing, detachment, or absence of emotional responsiveness

    (2) a reduction in awareness of his or her surroundings (e.g., "being in a daze")

    (3) derealization

    (4) depersonalization

    (5) dissociative amnesia (i.e., inability to recall an important aspect of the trauma)

C. The traumatic event is persistently reexperienced in at least one of the following ways: recurrent images, thoughts, dreams, illusions, flashback episodes, or a sense of reliving the experience; or distress on exposure to reminders of the traumatic event.

D. Marked avoidance of stimuli that arouse recollections of the trauma (e.g., thoughts, feelings, conversations, activities, places, people).

E. Marked symptoms of anxiety or increased arousal (e.g., difficulty sleeping, irritability, poor concentration, hypervigilance, exaggerated startle response, motor restlessness).

F. The disturbance causes clinically significant distress or impairment in social, occupational, or other important areas of functioning or impairs the individual's ability to pursue some necessary task, such as obtaining necessary assistance or mobilizing personal resources by telling family members about the traumatic experience.

**TABLE 4–14.   DSM-IV-TR criteria for acute stress
disorder (continued)**

G. The disturbance lasts for a minimum of 2 days and a maximum of
    4 weeks and occurs within 4 weeks of the traumatic event.

H. The disturbance is not due to the direct physiological effects of a
    substance (e.g., a drug of abuse, a medication) or a general medical
    condition, is not better accounted for by brief psychotic disorder, and
    is not merely an exacerbation of a preexisting Axis I or Axis II disorder.

---

and improving sleep, but their efficacy has not been established. Cognitive-behavioral therapies have been shown to help speed recovery and may even prevent PTSD when therapy is given over a few sessions beginning 2–3 weeks after trauma exposure.

Specific Phobia

A phobia is fear cued by a specific object or situation, which almost always provokes an immediate anxiety response or panic attack even though the patient recognizes that the fear is excessive or unreasonable. The phobic stimulus is avoided or endured with marked distress. The fear is usually not of the object, situation, or activity itself, but of some dreadful consequence that the patient believes may result from contact with the object, situation, or activity.

In DSM-IV-TR, specific phobia is subtyped on the basis of the object feared: natural environment (e.g., storms, water); animals (e.g., insects); blood, injection, or injury; situations (e.g., being in cars, airplanes, or tunnels); and other (e.g., choking, vomiting, or contracting an illness). The diagnostic criteria for specific phobia are shown in Table 4–15.

Differential Diagnosis

Specific phobias are usually not difficult to diagnose. However, the presence of other disorders that may cause irrational fears and avoidance behaviors should be ruled out.

Treatment

Medications do not appear to be useful in treating specific phobias. In contrast, exposure therapies have been shown to be efficacious in treat-

---

TABLE 4–15. DSM-IV-TR criteria for specific phobia

A. Marked and persistent fear that is excessive or unreasonable, cued by the presence or anticipation of a specific object or situation (e.g., flying, heights, animals, receiving an injection, seeing blood).

B. Exposure to the phobic stimulus almost invariably provokes an immediate anxiety response, which may take the form of a situationally bound or situationally predisposed panic attack. **Note:** In children, the anxiety may be expressed by crying, tantrums, freezing, or clinging.

C. The person recognizes that the fear is excessive or unreasonable. **Note:** In children, this feature may be absent.

D. The phobic situation(s) is avoided or else is endured with intense anxiety or distress.

E. The avoidance, anxious anticipation, or distress in the feared situation(s) interferes significantly with the person's normal routine, occupational (or academic) functioning, or social activities or relationships, or there is marked distress about having the phobia.

F. In individuals under age 18 years, the duration is at least 6 months.

G. The anxiety, panic attacks, or phobic avoidance associated with the specific object or situation are not better accounted for by another mental disorder, such as obsessive-compulsive disorder (e.g., fear of dirt in someone with an obsession about contamination), posttraumatic stress disorder (e.g., avoidance of stimuli associated with a severe stressor), separation anxiety disorder (e.g., avoidance of school), social phobia (e.g., avoidance of social situations because of fear of embarrassment), panic disorder with agoraphobia, or agoraphobia without history of panic disorder.

Specify type:

Animal type

Natural environment type (e.g., heights, storms, water)

Blood-injection-injury type

Situational type (e.g., airplanes, elevators, enclosed places)

Other type (e.g., fear of choking, vomiting, or contracting an illness; in children, fear of loud sounds or costumed characters)

---

ing specific phobia. In vivo exposure involves live exposure to the phobic object and is usually conducted in a graded fashion. Systematic desensitization uses progressive muscle relaxation to manage anxiety during imagined exposure to the phobic stimulus.

Social Phobia

In social phobia, patients have a persistent fear that they will humiliate or embarrass themselves in front of others. These patients usually avoid a variety of situations in which they may have to interact with others. Typical avoidance situations include speaking and eating in public, using public restrooms, and attending social gatherings or interviews. Somatic symptoms such as blushing and dry mouth are common in social phobia. Many patients "self-medicate" with alcohol and sedative drugs to alleviate the anticipatory anxiety related to this disorder. Actual panic attacks may also occur in persons with social phobia, and it may be difficult to distinguish between social phobia and agoraphobia when social avoidance accompanies panic attacks. The DSM-IV-TR diagnostic criteria for social phobia are shown in Table 4–16.

Differential Diagnosis

The avoidance associated with social phobia can also be seen in other disorders, such as agoraphobia, OCD, depressive disorders, schizophrenia, and paranoid disorders (Table 4–17). Some patients with agoraphobia are worried they will embarrass themselves while in a social setting, but unlike patients with social phobia, these patients experience panic attacks that occur in situations not involving evaluation by others.

Treatment

SSRIs have become first-line treatment for social phobia. Benzodiazepines have also been shown to be effective but are not considered first-line because of abuse potential. For performance-type social phobia, beta-blockers can be effective when used before a performance. The most commonly used beta-blockers for this purpose are propranolol (20 mg) or atenolol (50 mg), taken about 45 minutes before a performance.

TABLE 4–16. DSM-IV-TR criteria for social phobia

A. A marked and persistent fear of one or more social or performance situations in which the person is exposed to unfamiliar people or to possible scrutiny by others. The individual fears that he or she will act in a way (or show anxiety symptoms) that will be humiliating or embarrassing. **Note:** In children, there must be evidence of the capacity for age-appropriate social relationships with familiar people and the anxiety must occur in peer settings, not just in interactions with adults.

B. Exposure to the feared social situation almost invariably provokes anxiety, which may take the form of a situationally bound or situationally predisposed panic attack. **Note:** In children, the anxiety may be expressed by crying, tantrums, freezing, or shrinking from social situations with unfamiliar people.

C. The person recognizes that the fear is excessive or unreasonable. **Note:** In children, this feature may be absent.

D. The feared social or performance situations are avoided or else are endured with intense anxiety or distress.

E. The avoidance, anxious anticipation, or distress in the feared social or performance situation(s) interferes significantly with the person's normal routine, occupational (academic) functioning, or social activities or relationships, or there is marked distress about having the phobia.

F. In individuals under age 18 years, the duration is at least 6 months.

G. The fear or avoidance is not due to the direct physiological effects of a substance (e.g., a drug of abuse, a medication) or a general medical condition and is not better accounted for by another mental disorder (e.g., panic disorder with or without agoraphobia, separation anxiety disorder, body dysmorphic disorder, a pervasive developmental disorder, or schizoid personality disorder).

H. If a general medical condition or another mental disorder is present, the fear in criterion A is unrelated to it, e.g., the fear is not of stuttering, trembling in Parkinson's disease, or exhibiting abnormal eating behavior in anorexia nervosa or bulimia nervosa.

Specify if:

Generalized: if the fears include most social situations (also consider the additional diagnosis of avoidant personality disorder)

TABLE 4–17.   Differential diagnosis of social phobia

Personality disorder, such as avoidant, schizoid, paranoid

Axis I paranoid disorder, such as paranoid schizophrenia or paranoid delusional disorder

Depression-related social withdrawal secondary to anhedonia or feelings of defectiveness

Obsessive-compulsive disorder–related fears exacerbated in social settings (e.g., contamination)

Panic disorder with phobic avoidance not limited to social situations

Deficits or impaired social skills associated with schizophrenia and related disorders

Body dysmorphic disorder with secondary social phobia

Source.   Adapted from Hales and Yudofsky 2003.

References

American Psychiatric Association: Diagnostic and Statistical Manual of Mental Disorders, 4th Edition, Text Revision. Washington, DC, American Psychiatric Association, 2000

Hales RE, Yudofsky SC: The American Psychiatric Publishing Textbook of Clinical Psychiatry, 4th Edition. Washington, DC, American Psychiatric Publishing, 2003

Jenike MA: Approaches to the patient with treatment-refractory obsessive compulsive disorder. J Clin Psychiatry 51(suppl):15–21, 1990

Kessler RC, Berglund P, Demler O, et al: Lifetime prevalence and age-of-onset distributions of DSM-IV disorders in the National Comorbidity Survey Replication. Arch Gen Psychiatry 62:593–602, 2005a

Kessler RC, Chiu WT, Demler O, et al: Prevalence, severity, and comorbidity of 12-month DSM-IV disorders in the National Comorbidity Survey Replication. Arch Gen Psychiatry 62:617–627, 2005b

Raskind MA, Peskind ER, Hoff DJ, et al: A parallel group placebo controlled study of prazosin for trauma nightmares and sleep disturbance in combat veterans with post-traumatic stress disorder. Biol Psychiatry 61:928–934, 2007

5

Personality Disorders

Personality disorders are characterized by enduring maladaptive patterns of perceiving, relating to, and thinking about the environment, other people, and oneself. A personality disorder is diagnosed when personality traits become inflexible and pervasive to the point where they cause significant social or occupational dysfunction, or subjective distress.

Key Points

- Personality features must be present by early adulthood.
- Diagnosis typically requires multiple assessments over time.
- Behaviors are often quite distressing and problematic for both the patients and those close to them.
- Diagnosis requires consideration of the individual's ethnic, cultural, and social background.
- Personality disorders are coded on Axis II.
- Mixed personality disorder is probably the most common form of personality disorder. It is usually coded personality disorder not otherwise specified (NOS), with the specific features (narcissistic, self-defeating, histrionic) listed (G.O. Gabbard, personal communication, August 2007).

Clusters

Personality disorders are grouped into three clusters, although patients may present with comorbidity across clusters. Table 5–1 shows the prevalence of personality disorders by cluster.

- Cluster A: Patients often appear odd or eccentric; includes paranoid, schizoid, and schizotypal personality disorders.
- Cluster B: Patients often appear dramatic, emotional, or erratic; includes antisocial, borderline, histrionic, and narcissistic personality disorders.
- Cluster C: Patients often appear anxious or fearful; includes avoidant, dependent, and obsessive-compulsive personality disorders.

The DSM-IV-TR (American Psychiatric Association 2000) general diagnostic criteria for a personality disorder are outlined in Table 5–2. Each personality disorder has additional, specific criteria, which are outlined in the appropriate subsection of this chapter.

General Treatment for Patients With Personality Disorders

In general, psychotherapy is the treatment of choice for personality disorders (see Table 5–3). Medications may be useful for the treatment of specific symptom clusters. For example, antidepressants may be helpful if the patient suffers from depressive and anxiety symptoms. Antipsychotic medications may be appropriate if the patient presents with delusional thinking.

Paranoid Personality Disorder

Key feature: Chronic distrust and unjustified suspicion of others.

Table 5–4 presents the full diagnostic criteria for paranoid personality disorder.

Differential Diagnosis

- Patients with paranoid personality disorder differ from those with schizophrenia because they do not generally lose touch with reality or experience hallucinations.

TABLE 5–1. Prevalence of personality disorders in the National Comorbidity Survey Replication study

TYPE OF DISORDER	PREVALENCE
All personality disorders	9.1
Cluster A	5.7
Cluster B	1.5
Antisocial	0.6
Borderline	1.3
Cluster C	6.0

Source. Adapted from Lenzenweger et al. 2007.

TABLE 5–2. DSM-IV-TR general diagnostic criteria for a personality disorder

A. An enduring pattern of inner experience and behavior that deviates markedly from the expectations of the individual's culture. This pattern is manifested in two (or more) of the following areas:

(1) cognition (i.e., ways of perceiving and interpreting self, other people, and events)

(2) affectivity (i.e., the range, intensity, lability, and appropriateness of emotional response)

(3) interpersonal functioning

(4) impulse control

B. The enduring pattern is inflexible and pervasive across a broad range of personal and social situations.

C. The enduring pattern leads to clinically significant distress or impairment in social, occupational, or other important areas of functioning.

D. The pattern is stable and of long duration, and its onset can be traced back at least to adolescence or early adulthood.

E. The enduring pattern is not better accounted for as a manifestation or consequence of another mental disorder.

F. The enduring pattern is not due to the direct physiological effects of a substance (e.g., a drug of abuse, a medication) or a general medical condition (e.g., head trauma).

TABLE 5–3. Evidence of treatment effectiveness for personality disorders

PERSONALITY DISORDER	PSYCHOTHERAPIES	PSYCHOSOCIAL THERAPIES	PHARMACOTHERAPIES
Paranoid	–	–	±
Schizoid	+	+	–
Schizotypal	–	±	+
Antisocial	–	+	–
Borderline	+	++	+
Histrionic	++	–	–
Narcissistic	++	–	–
Avoidant	++	+	±
Dependent	++	+	–
Obsessive-compulsive	++	–	–

Note.   –=no support; ±=uncertain support; +=moderately helpful; ++=significantly helpful.
Source.   Adapted from Hales and Yudofsky 2004.

- Patients with paranoid personality disorder can be differentiated from the other Cluster A disorders in that they are not indifferent to others, as seen in schizoid personality disorder, and they do not experience magical thinking or odd speech, as seen in schizotypal personality disorder.
- It is important to rule out medical disorders and substance-induced conditions if the personality changes are temporally related to either the onset of a medical disorder or the use of drugs or medication.

Treatment

- Individuals with paranoid personality disorder do not typically seek treatment.
- Antipsychotic medication and supportive therapy may be helpful, if symptoms are severe.

TABLE 5–4. DSM-IV-TR criteria for paranoid personality disorder

A. A pervasive distrust and suspiciousness of others such that their motives are interpreted as malevolent, beginning by early adulthood and present in a variety of contexts, as indicated by four (or more) of the following:

   (1) suspects, without sufficient basis, that others are exploiting, harming, or deceiving him or her

   (2) is preoccupied with unjustified doubts about the loyalty or trustworthiness of friends or associates

   (3) is reluctant to confide in others because of unwarranted fear that the information will be used maliciously against him or her

   (4) reads hidden demeaning or threatening meanings into benign remarks or events

   (5) persistently bears grudges, i.e., is unforgiving of insults, injuries, or slights

   (6) perceives attacks on his or her character or reputation that are not apparent to others and is quick to react angrily or to counterattack

   (7) has recurrent suspicions, without justification, regarding fidelity of spouse or sexual partner

B. Does not occur exclusively during the course of schizophrenia, a mood disorder with psychotic features, or another psychotic disorder and is not due to the direct physiological effects of a general medical condition.
   Note: If criteria are met prior to the onset of schizophrenia, add "premorbid," e.g., "paranoid personality disorder (premorbid)."

Schizoid Personality Disorder

Key feature: Ego-syntonic detachment from social relationships.

   Table 5–5 presents the full diagnostic criteria for schizoid personality disorder.

Differential Diagnosis

- Patients with this disorder may appear to have negative symptoms of schizophrenia, but they do not typically experience the positive symptoms (e.g., delusions and hallucinations).

TABLE 5–5.   DSM-IV-TR criteria for schizoid personality disorder

---

A. A pervasive pattern of detachment from social relationships and a restricted range of expression of emotions in interpersonal settings, beginning by early adulthood and present in a variety of contexts, as indicated by four (or more) of the following:

   (1) neither desires nor enjoys close relationships, including being part of a family

   (2) almost always chooses solitary activities

   (3) has little, if any, interest in having sexual experiences with another person

   (4) takes pleasure in few, if any, activities

   (5) lacks close friends or confidants other than first-degree relatives

   (6) appears indifferent to the praise or criticism of others

   (7) shows emotional coldness, detachment, or flattened affectivity

B. Does not occur exclusively during the course of schizophrenia, a mood disorder with psychotic features, another psychotic disorder, or a pervasive developmental disorder and is not due to the direct physiological effects of a general medical condition.
   Note: If criteria are met prior to the onset of schizophrenia, add "premorbid," e.g., "schizoid personality disorder (premorbid)."

- They may also appear to have avoidant personality disorder, because they avoid interactions with others, but they do not exhibit the fear of criticism and rejection evident in patients with avoidant personality disorder.

- This disorder can be differentiated from other Cluster A disorders in that these patients do not have suspiciousness as seen in paranoid personality disorder or cognitive and perceptual distortions as seen in schizotypal personality disorder.

- It is important to rule out medical disorders and substance-induced conditions if the personality changes are temporally related to either the onset of a medical disorder or the intake of drugs or medication.

Treatment

- Patients with schizoid personality disorder do not typically seek treatment unless they are under increased stress in their life or a friend or family member insists on treatment.
- Brief, solution-focused therapy approaches may be the most helpful. Cognitive-behavioral therapy may also be appropriate to target certain types of irrational thoughts that are negatively influencing the patient's behaviors.
- Stability and support are important aspects in treating patients with schizoid personality disorder.
- Comorbid disorders (e.g., depression) should be treated.

Schizotypal Personality Disorder

Key features: Odd behaviors, inappropriate responses to social cues, and peculiar beliefs.

Table 5–6 presents the full diagnostic criteria for schizotypal personality disorder.

Differential Diagnosis

- Patients with schizotypal personality disorder do not experience the frank delusions and hallucinations typically seen in schizophrenia, but they may experience brief periods of psychosis.
- As with the other Cluster A disorders, it is important to rule out medical disorders and substance-induced conditions if the personality changes are temporally related to either the onset of a medical disorder or the intake of drugs or medication.

Treatment

- Behavioral therapies, with an emphasis on social skills training, that focus on the basics of social relationships and social interactions may be beneficial.
- Medication may be useful during acute phases of psychosis, which are likely to manifest themselves during times of extreme stress or difficult life events.
- Small case series have reported on the effectiveness of low-dose antipsychotic medications to help with the anxiety and psychosis associated with this disorder (Goldberg et al. 1986).

TABLE 5–6.   DSM-IV-TR criteria for schizotypal personality disorder

---

A. A pervasive pattern of social and interpersonal deficits marked by acute discomfort with, and reduced capacity for, close relationships as well as by cognitive or perceptual distortions and eccentricities of behavior, beginning by early adulthood and present in a variety of contexts, as indicated by five (or more) of the following:

   (1) ideas of reference (excluding delusions of reference)

   (2) odd beliefs or magical thinking that influences behavior and is inconsistent with subcultural norms (e.g., superstitiousness, belief in clairvoyance, telepathy, or "sixth sense"; in children and adolescents, bizarre fantasies or preoccupations)

   (3) unusual perceptual experiences, including bodily illusions

   (4) odd thinking and speech (e.g., vague, circumstantial, metaphorical, overelaborate, or stereotyped)

   (5) suspiciousness or paranoid ideation

   (6) inappropriate or constricted affect

   (7) behavior or appearance that is odd, eccentric, or peculiar

   (8) lack of close friends or confidants other than first-degree relatives

   (9) excessive social anxiety that does not diminish with familiarity and tends to be associated with paranoid fears rather than negative judgments about self

B. Does not occur exclusively during the course of schizophrenia, a mood disorder with psychotic features, another psychotic disorder, or a pervasive developmental disorder.
   Note: If criteria are met prior to the onset of schizophrenia, add "premorbid," e.g., "schizotypal personality disorder (premorbid)."

Antisocial Personality Disorder

Key features: Long-standing disregard for other people's rights; a pervasive lack of remorse.

The pattern of behavior must be present since age 15, but the personality disorder cannot be diagnosed until the patient is at least 18 years old. Table 5–7 presents the full diagnostic criteria for antisocial personality disorder.

TABLE 5–7. DSM-IV-TR criteria for antisocial personality disorder

A. There is a pervasive pattern of disregard for and violation of the rights of others occurring since age 15 years, as indicated by three (or more) of the following:

 (1) failure to conform to social norms with respect to lawful behaviors as indicated by repeatedly performing acts that are grounds for arrest

 (2) deceitfulness, as indicated by repeated lying, use of aliases, or conning others for personal profit or pleasure

 (3) impulsivity or failure to plan ahead

 (4) irritability and aggressiveness, as indicated by repeated physical fights or assaults

 (5) reckless disregard for safety of self or others

 (6) consistent irresponsibility, as indicated by repeated failure to sustain consistent work behavior or honor financial obligations

 (7) lack of remorse, as indicated by being indifferent to or rationalizing having hurt, mistreated, or stolen from another

B. The individual is at least age 18 years.

C. There is evidence of conduct disorder with onset before age 15 years.

D. The occurrence of antisocial behavior is not exclusively during the course of schizophrenia or a manic episode.

Differential Diagnosis

- Compared with the other personality disorders, antisocial personality disorder is usually less difficult to diagnose because of its characteristic pattern of behaviors.

- These patients may appear narcissistic, but patients with narcissistic personality disorder do not exhibit the impulsive or physically aggressive behaviors seen with antisocial personality disorder.

- Patients with histrionic personality disorder or borderline personality disorder (BPD) can appear impulsive and manipulative, but these patients are seeking attention and nurturance; patients with antisocial personality disorder are typically seeking power or material gain (Skodol 2005).

- During psychotic episodes or manic episodes, patients may commit antisocial acts. In these cases, the Axis I disorder preempts the personality disorder diagnosis.

Treatment

- Individual psychotherapy is the primary treatment of choice; however, these patients are typically not motivated to use psychotherapy.
- Patients with antisocial disorder can have a disruptive influence on treatment teams and other patients.
- Medications may help stabilize mood swings or specific and acute Axis I concurrent diagnoses.

Borderline Personality Disorder

Key feature: Instability in affect, identity, and impulse control.

Patients with BPD highly utilize psychiatric outpatient, inpatient, and psychopharmacological treatment (Bender et al. 2001). Comorbid disorders, such as substance use and mood disorders, are common in these patients. Table 5–8 presents the full diagnostic criteria for BPD.

Differential Diagnosis

- Some features of BPD may overlap with those of mood disorders, making it difficult to differentiate.
- In bipolar disorder, mood episodes generally last weeks or months. In BPD, marked emotional lability and mood reactivity typically occur in response to external stressors and may only last for seconds, minutes, hours, or days. However, these two disorders may co-occur. Thus, it is important to assess the symptoms over time.
- Patients with BPD may appear histrionic because of demanding and manipulative behaviors, but histrionic patients do not typically engage in self-destructive behaviors.

Treatment

- Pharmacological and cognitive-behavioral interventions are useful in the treatment of BPD (American Psychiatric Association 2001).

TABLE 5–8. DSM-IV-TR criteria for borderline personality disorder

A pervasive pattern of instability of interpersonal relationships, self-image, and affects, and marked impulsivity beginning by early adulthood and present in a variety of contexts, as indicated by five (or more) of the following:

(1) frantic efforts to avoid real or imagined abandonment. **Note:** Do not include suicidal or self-mutilating behavior covered in criterion 5.

(2) a pattern of unstable and intense interpersonal relationships characterized by alternating between extremes of idealization and devaluation

(3) identity disturbance: markedly and persistently unstable self-image or sense of self

(4) impulsivity in at least two areas that are potentially self-damaging (e.g., spending, sex, substance abuse, reckless driving, binge eating). **Note:** Do not include suicidal or self-mutilating behavior covered in criterion 5.

(5) recurrent suicidal behavior, gestures, or threats, or self-mutilating behavior

(6) affective instability due to a marked reactivity of mood (e.g., intense episodic dysphoria, irritability, or anxiety usually lasting a few hours and only rarely more than a few days)

(7) chronic feelings of emptiness

(8) inappropriate, intense anger or difficulty controlling anger (e.g., frequent displays of temper, constant anger, recurrent physical fights)

(9) transient, stress-related paranoid ideation or severe dissociative symptoms

- Dialectical behavior therapy has been shown to significantly reduce self-injury and suicidal behavior in patients with BPD (Linehan et al. 2006; see also Chapter 15, "Psychotherapy and Psychosocial Treatments").

- Medications may help alleviate impulsivity, affective lability, irritability and aggressive behavior (Coccaro and Kavoussi 1997). Most published studies have used selective serotonin reuptake inhibitors, which have become the treatment of choice.

Histrionic Personality Disorder

Key features: Excessive emotionality; attention-seeking behavior.

Patients with histrionic personality disorder often come across as "fake" or shallow in their interpersonal relationships with others. Table 5–9 presents the full diagnostic criteria for histrionic personality disorder.

Differential Diagnosis

- Patients with histrionic personality disorder may appear narcissistic in their attention seeking, but they will often seem weak or dependent in an attempt to attract attention; someone with narcissistic personality disorder usually seeks attention for superiority and power.
- These patients share some characteristics with BPD, but they do not exhibit the self-destructiveness associated with BPD.

Treatment

- Individual psychodynamic psychotherapy

TABLE 5–9.   DSM-IV-TR criteria for histrionic personality disorder

---

A pervasive pattern of excessive emotionality and attention seeking, beginning by early adulthood and present in a variety of contexts, as indicated by five (or more) of the following:

(1) is uncomfortable in situations in which he or she is not the center of attention

(2) interaction with others is often characterized by inappropriate sexually seductive or provocative behavior

(3) displays rapidly shifting and shallow expression of emotions

(4) consistently uses physical appearance to draw attention to self

(5) has a style of speech that is excessively impressionistic and lacking in detail

(6) shows self-dramatization, theatricality, and exaggerated expression of emotion

(7) is suggestible, i.e., easily influenced by others or circumstances

(8) considers relationships to be more intimate than they actually are

---

Narcissistic Personality Disorder

Key features: Grandiose sense of self; a need for admiration.

Patients with narcissistic personality disorder often seek out and feel entitled to see the most senior physician in a prestigious institution. Table 5–10 presents the full diagnostic criteria for narcissistic personality disorder.

Differential Diagnosis

- A patient with narcissistic personality disorder may present with Axis I symptoms and disorders at various times in his or her life.
- Some characteristics of this disorder overlap with other Cluster B disorders, as described earlier in this chapter.
- These patients may seem perfectionistic, but they differ from patients with obsessive-compulsive personality disorder because they are not self-critical.

Treatment

- Individual psychodynamic psychotherapy

Avoidant Personality Disorder

Key features: Feelings of inadequacy, fear of negative evaluation by others, and social inhibition.

These patients typically have poor self-esteem and may have difficulty looking at situations and interactions in an objective manner. Table 5–11 presents the full diagnostic criteria for avoidant personality disorder.

Differential Diagnosis

- Avoidant personality disorder shares features with dependent personality disorder, but patients with the former disorder are not as concerned about being taken care of as are patients with the latter disorder.
- Avoidant personality disorder may be difficult to distinguish from social phobia, and these two disorders often co-occur. However, avoidant personality disorder involves feelings of inade-

---

TABLE 5–10. DSM-IV-TR criteria for narcissistic personality disorder

---

A pervasive pattern of grandiosity (in fantasy or behavior), need for admiration, and lack of empathy, beginning by early adulthood and present in a variety of contexts, as indicated by five (or more) of the following:

(1) has a grandiose sense of self-importance (e.g., exaggerates achievements and talents, expects to be recognized as superior without commensurate achievements)

(2) is preoccupied with fantasies of unlimited success, power, brilliance, beauty, or ideal love

(3) believes that he or she is "special" and unique and can only be understood by, or should associate with, other special or high-status people (or institutions)

(4) requires excessive admiration

(5) has a sense of entitlement, i.e., unreasonable expectations of especially favorable treatment or automatic compliance with his or her expectations

(6) is interpersonally exploitative, i.e., takes advantage of others to achieve his or her own ends

(7) lacks empathy: is unwilling to recognize or identify with the feelings and needs of others

(8) is often envious of others or believes that others are envious of him or her

(9) shows arrogant, haughty behaviors or attitudes

---

quacy and inferiority, whereas social phobia consists of specific fears related to social performance.

- Schizoid personality disorder involves social isolation, but these patients do not want relationships, whereas patients with avoidant personality disorder desire relationships but fear them.

Treatment

- Individual psychotherapy oriented toward finding solutions to specific life problems
- Assertiveness and social skills training

TABLE 5–11.   DSM-IV-TR criteria for avoidant personality disorder

A pervasive pattern of social inhibition, feelings of inadequacy, and hypersensitivity to negative evaluation, beginning by early adulthood and present in a variety of contexts, as indicated by four (or more) of the following:

(1) avoids occupational activities that involve significant interpersonal contact, because of fears of criticism, disapproval, or rejection

(2) is unwilling to get involved with people unless certain of being liked

(3) shows restraint within intimate relationships because of the fear of being shamed or ridiculed

(4) is preoccupied with being criticized or rejected in social situations

(5) is inhibited in new interpersonal situations because of feelings of inadequacy

(6) views self as socially inept, personally unappealing, or inferior to others

(7) is unusually reluctant to take personal risks or to engage in any new activities because they may prove embarrassing

Dependent Personality Disorder

Key features: An excessive need to be taken care of; submissive behaviors.

Patients with dependent personality disorder often present with depression and anxiety symptoms, as well as a number of physical or somatic complaints. Table 5–12 presents the full diagnostic criteria for dependent personality disorder.

Differential Diagnosis

- Dependent personality disorder often co-occurs with other personality disorders, especially avoidant personality disorder.
- Significant distress or social or occupational dysfunction is required for the diagnosis and is important in the differential diagnosis.

Treatment

- Individual psychotherapy is directed toward increasing the patient's self-esteem, sense of effectiveness, assertiveness, and independent functioning.
- Couples or family therapy may be useful if the patient is in a relationship that is maintaining or reinforcing the dependent behavior.

TABLE 5–12.   DSM-IV-TR criteria for dependent personality disorder

---

A pervasive and excessive need to be taken care of that leads to submissive and clinging behavior and fears of separation, beginning by early adulthood and present in a variety of contexts, as indicated by five (or more) of the following:

(1) has difficulty making everyday decisions without an excessive amount of advice and reassurance from others

(2) needs others to assume responsibility for most major areas of his or her life

(3) has difficulty expressing disagreement with others because of fear of loss of support or approval. **Note:** Do not include realistic fears of retribution.

(4) has difficulty initiating projects or doing things on his or her own (because of a lack of self-confidence in judgment or abilities rather than a lack of motivation or energy)

(5) goes to excessive lengths to obtain nurturance and support from others, to the point of volunteering to do things that are unpleasant

(6) feels uncomfortable or helpless when alone because of exaggerated fears of being unable to care for himself or herself

(7) urgently seeks another relationship as a source of care and support when a close relationship ends

(8) is unrealistically preoccupied with fears of being left to take care of himself or herself

---

Obsessive-Compulsive Personality Disorder

Key features: Perfectionism; inflexibility; being overly controlling.

Patients with obsessive-compulsive personality disorder may seem difficult to treat because of their excessive intellectualizations and difficulty expressing emotions. Table 5–13 presents the full diagnostic criteria for obsessive-compulsive personality disorder.

TABLE 5–13. DSM-IV-TR criteria for obsessive-compulsive personality disorder

---

A pervasive pattern of preoccupation with orderliness, perfectionism, and mental and interpersonal control, at the expense of flexibility, openness, and efficiency, beginning by early adulthood and present in a variety of contexts, as indicated by four (or more) of the following:

(1) is preoccupied with details, rules, lists, order, organization, or schedules to the extent that the major point of the activity is lost

(2) shows perfectionism that interferes with task completion (e.g., is unable to complete a project because his or her own overly strict standards are not met)

(3) is excessively devoted to work and productivity to the exclusion of leisure activities and friendships (not accounted for by obvious economic necessity)

(4) is overconscientious, scrupulous, and inflexible about matters of morality, ethics, or values (not accounted for by cultural or religious identification)

(5) is unable to discard worn-out or worthless objects even when they have no sentimental value

(6) is reluctant to delegate tasks or to work with others unless they submit to exactly his or her way of doing things

(7) adopts a miserly spending style toward both self and others; money is viewed as something to be hoarded for future catastrophes

(8) shows rigidity and stubbornness

Differential Diagnosis

- Obsessive-compulsive disorder is an anxiety disorder that is not necessarily associated with a need for order, whereas obsessive-compulsive personality disorder is typically ego-syntonic and not associated with intrusive ego-dystonic thoughts.

Treatment

- Individual psychotherapy, group psychotherapy, and behavioral techniques have all been described as useful in the treatment of obsessive-compulsive personality disorder.

References

American Psychiatric Association: Diagnostic and Statistical Manual of Mental Disorders, 4th Edition, Text Revision. Washington, DC, American Psychiatric Association, 2000

American Psychiatric Association: Practice guideline for the treatment of patients with borderline personality disorder. Am J Psychiatry 158(suppl):1–52, 2001

Bender DS, Dolan RT, Skodol AE, et al: Treatment utilization by patients with personality disorders. Am J Psychiatry 158:295–302, 2001

Coccaro EF, Kavoussi RJ: Fluoxetine and impulsive aggressive behavior in personality-disordered subjects. Arch Gen Psychiatry 54:1081–1088, 1997

Goldberg SC, Schulz C, Schulz PM, et al: Borderline and schizotypal personality disorders treated with low-dose thiothixene vs placebo. Arch Gen Psychiatry 43:680–686, 1986

Hales RE, Yudofsky SC: Essentials of Clinical Psychiatry, 2nd Edition. Washington, DC, American Psychiatric Publishing, 2004

Lenzenweger MF, Lane MC, Loranger AW, et al: DSM-IV personality disorders in the National Comorbidity Survey replication. Biol Psychiatry 62:553–564, 2007

Linehan MM, Comtois KA, Murray AM, et al: Two-year randomized controlled trial and follow-up of dialectical behavior therapy vs. therapy by experts for suicidal behaviors and borderline personality disorder. Arch Gen Psychiatry 63:757–766, 2006

Skodol AE: Manifestations, clinical diagnosis, and comorbidity, in The American Psychiatric Publishing Textbook of Personality Disorders. Edited by Oldham JM, Skodol AE, Bender DS. Washington, DC, American Psychiatric Publishing, 2005

6

Sleep Disorders

Insomnia

The key feature of insomnia is difficulty initiating and maintaining duration or quality of sleep that interferes with daily function, despite adequate opportunity and environment to achieve sleep.

- Transient insomnia occurs for less than 1 week.
- Short-term insomnia occurs for 1–4 weeks.
- Chronic insomnia is present for more than 1 month.

The prevalence of insomnia is 10%–15%. A higher incidence of insomnia is seen in

- Women,
- Older people,
- People with psychiatric disorders, and
- People with chronic medical conditions.

Table 6–1 presents the DSM-IV-TR (American Psychiatric Association 2000) criteria for primary insomnia.

Classifications

PRIMARY INSOMNIA

- Idiopathic
- Psychophysiological or learned insomnia

TABLE 6–1.   DSM-IV-TR criteria for primary insomnia

A. The predominant complaint is difficulty initiating or maintaining sleep, or nonrestorative sleep, for at least 1 month.

B. The sleep disturbance (or associated daytime fatigue) causes clinically significant distress or impairment in social, occupational, or other important areas of functioning.

C. The sleep disturbance does not occur exclusively during the course of narcolepsy, breathing-related sleep disorder, circadian rhythm sleep disorder, or a parasomnia.

D. The disturbance does not occur exclusively during the course of another mental disorder (e.g., major depressive disorder, generalized anxiety disorder, a delirium).

E. The disturbance is not due to the direct physiological effects of a substance (e.g., a drug of abuse, a medication) or a general medical condition.

- Paradoxical insomnia or sleep state misperception
- Behavioral insomnia of childhood secondary to reliance on external soothing devices (bottle or pacifier) and refusal to go to bed

SECONDARY INSOMNIA

- Adjustment insomnia secondary to life events or stress
- Insomnia secondary to poor sleep habits, such as inconsistent sleep times.
- Insomnia secondary to psychiatric disease, specifically depression or anxiety
- Insomnia secondary to medical conditions (e.g., chronic pain, hot flashes)
- Insomnia secondary to medication side effects (e.g., alcohol, steroids, caffeine)

Treatment

- Eliminate untreated conditions such as depression, pain sources, and urinary urgency. Initiate cognitive-behavioral therapy (described later in this section).

- If no response, initiate medication, adjusting the dose for elderly patients and patients with comorbid disease (e.g., no benzodiazepines for patients with severe obstructive sleep apnea [OSA]). Long-term use of hypnotics is off-label.

Pharmacotherapy options include ramelteon and nonbenzodiazepine hypnotics (see Table 6–2; see also Chapter 14, "Pharmacotherapy"). Ramelteon is a melatonin MT_1 and MT_2 receptor agonist with a half-life of 1–2.6 hours; studies show decreased sleep latency (Roth et al. 2006a).

Cognitive-behavioral therapy techniques include the following:

- Stimulus control therapy: Reestablish the bed as the place where sleep happens, rather than the site of sleeplessness.
- Paradoxical intention: Patients are encouraged to deliberately intensify symptoms of insomnia in order to increase awareness of these symptoms and their consequences.
- Sleep restriction: Restrict sleeping time to reduce the time spent awake in bed and to establish new sleep routines.
- Relaxation.

Narcolepsy

Narcolepsy is excessive daytime sleepiness with one of the following: cataplexy, sleep paralysis, hallucinations, or sleep fragmentation. Table 6–3 presents the DSM-IV-TR diagnostic criteria for narcolepsy.

TABLE 6–2.   Nonbenzodiazepine hypnotics

DRUG	**DOSE (MG)**	**GERIATRIC DOSE (MG)**	**HALF-LIFE (HOURS)**
Zaleplon (Sonata)	5–10	5	1
Zolpidem (Ambien)	5–10	5	1.5–5
Zolpidem controlled-release (Ambien CR)	6.25–12.5	6.25	4–5
Eszopiclone (Lunesta)	2–3	1–2	6

Source.   Adapted from Marangell and Martinez 2006.

TABLE 6–3.   DSM-IV-TR criteria for narcolepsy

A. Irresistible attacks of refreshing sleep that occur daily over at least 3 months.

B. The presence of one or both of the following:

(1) cataplexy (i.e., brief episodes of sudden bilateral loss of muscle tone, most often in association with intense emotion)

(2) recurrent intrusions of elements of rapid eye movement (REM) sleep into the transition between sleep and wakefulness, as manifested by either hypnopompic or hypnagogic hallucinations or sleep paralysis at the beginning or end of sleep episodes

C. The disturbance is not due to the direct physiological effects of a substance (e.g., a drug of abuse, a medication) or another general medical condition.

- *Cataplexy* is the suppression of skeletal muscle activity (excluding eye and diaphragmatic muscles) that occurs outside of rapid eye movement (REM) sleep. It is frequently induced by strong emotion, particularly humor or laughter.

- *Sleep paralysis* is muscle paralysis that occurs on wakening.

- *Hypnagogic (onset-of-sleep)* and *hypnopompic (end-of-sleep) hallucinations* are dreamlike and occur during the transition between sleep and wakefulness.

- *Sleep fragmentation* is a polysomnography observation that reveals increase in shifting between sleep stages, low sleep efficiency, and a decrease in slow wave sleep, stages 3 and 4.

The prevalence of narcolepsy is 1:2,000, with men and women equally affected. Onset is usually before age 25 years. The disorder is underdiagnosed. It is a chronic illness without cure, requiring chronic treatment.

Differential Diagnosis

- Depression
- Epilepsy
- OSA
- Sleep deprivation

- Chronic fatigue syndrome
- Hyperthyroidism
- Drug abuse
- Periodic limb movement disorder (PLMD)
- Idiopathic hypersomnia
- Kleine-Levin syndrome

Assessment

- Overnight polysomnogram followed by multiple sleep latency test (MSLT). If the overnight polysomnogram reveals alternative etiology for excessive daytime somnolence (e.g., OSA or PLMD), treatment must be adequate for the OSA or the PLMD prior to the diagnostic MSLT for narcolepsy.
- Thyroid profile
- Complete blood count
- Magnetic resonance imaging (MRI) if there is suspicion of secondary causes, such as multiple sclerosis plaques in the hypothalamus or ischemic lesions in the hypothalamus
- Cerebrospinal fluid hypocretin-1 level if the MSLT is equivocal or inconsistent with clinical course

Treatment

- Sleep hygiene tactics
- Avoidance of shift work
- Regular timing of nocturnal sleep
- Timed 15-minute naps at midmorning, lunchtime, and late afternoon
- Educating and informing teachers, family, and employers of the need for naps to treat this disabling disease and prevent falls or accidents and improve productivity
- Pharmacological treatment of excessive daytime sleepiness
  - Dextroamphetamine
  - γ-Hydroxybutyric acid (GHB)
  - Methylphenidate
  - Methamphetamine
  - Mazindol

- Selegiline
- Modafinil
- Sodium oxybate

- Pharmacological treatment of cataplexy
  - Imipramine
  - Clomipramine
  - Desipramine
  - Protriptyline
  - Fluoxetine
  - Sodium oxybate
  - Venlafaxine
  - Atomoxetine

Breathing-Related Sleep Disorder

The incidence of breathing-related sleep disorder is 2%–5% of the general population. Table 6–4 presents the DSM-IV-TR diagnostic criteria for breathing-related sleep disorder.

Causes

Central sleep apnea is the absence of ventilatory effort. Ventilatory effort is triggered in the brain after sensing carbon dioxide (CO_2) levels at chemoreceptors. This feedback loop is impaired in diseases such as brainstem ischemia, autonomic dysfunction from diabetes, and congestive heart failure.

Obstructive sleep apnea (OSA) occurs as a result of impairment of mechanical flow. This impairment may result from obesity, congenitally narrow airway, tonsillar hypertrophy, nasal turbinate hypertrophy, abnormal mandibular position, or other causes.

- The clinical presentation of OSA includes complaints of daytime hypersomnolence, cognitive deficits, irritability, depression, decreased libido, and morning headaches; these symptoms are a result of the disruptive breathing at night and associated oxygen desaturation. Reports of disruptive snoring by the bed partner or family members are common.

TABLE 6–4. DSM-IV-TR criteria for breathing-related sleep
disorder

A. Sleep disruption, leading to excessive sleepiness or insomnia, that is
judged to be due to a sleep-related breathing condition (e.g.,
obstructive or central sleep apnea syndrome or central alveolar
hypoventilation syndrome).

B. The disturbance is not better accounted for by another mental
disorder and is not due to the direct physiological effects of a
substance (e.g., a drug of abuse, a medication) or another general
medical condition (other than a breathing-related disorder).

Coding note: Also code sleep-related breathing disorder on Axis III.

- Risk factors for OSA include older age, body mass index greater
  than 30 kg/m^2, supine sleeping, and a neck circumference greater
  than 17 inches. Alcohol or sedative intake prior to bedtime increases
  the risks.
- Long-term side effects of untreated OSA include an increase in
  the development of hypertension, myocardial infarction, and
  stroke (Buchner et al. 2007).

Treatment

- Weight loss to achieve optimal body mass index
- Sleeping in the lateral position
- Elevation of the head and trunk 30–60 degrees
- Abstaining from alcohol prior to bedtime
- Continuous positive airway pressure (CPAP) treatment is the
  most successful treatment used during all periods of sleep,
  including naps. CPAP is a pneumatic splinting of the airway to
  maintain upper-airway patency. This treatment requires commit-
  ment of the patient and physician to ensure proper mask fit and
  compliance; pharmacological intervention is needed to augment
  treatment. Modafinil and related compounds may improve daytime alertness in patients who are compliant with CPAP but continue to report daytime hypersomnolence (Roth et al. 2006b).
- Bi-level pressure may be necessary to accommodate patients with
  neuromuscular weakness or intolerance to continuous pressure.

Bi-level treatment allows the inspiratory pressure to be greater than the expiratory pressure while maintaining airway patency. This can best be determined in a laboratory setting.

- Dental appliances may improve mild disease. Decreased airway resistance results from advancing the mandible and tongue with the device.

- Surgical intervention is important for patients who cannot tolerate CPAP or who have difficulty optimizing CPAP secondary to airway resistance from nasal or palatal obstructions. These patients should be referred to an ear, nose, and throat specialist for tonsillectomy and adenoidectomy, resection of hypertrophied nasal turbinates, hyoid myotomy, or mandibular advancement as appropriate.

- The American Academy of Pediatrics recommends evaluation for tonsillectomy in children with persistent disruptive snoring (Schechter 2002).

Circadian Rhythm Sleep Disorder

Circadian rhythm sleep disorder is defined as a mismatch between sleep pattern and desired "normal" societal pattern. Table 6–5 presents the DSM-IV-TR diagnostic criteria for circadian rhythm sleep disorder.

- *Delayed sleep phase syndrome* occurs primarily in adolescents whose sleep and wake times are later than desired (e.g., initiation of sleep at 2 A.M. and wakening at 10 A.M.). These patients should minimize exposure to light before bedtime.

- *Advanced sleep phase syndrome* occurs predominantly in older patients whose sleep and wake times occur earlier than desired (e.g., sleep initiation at 7 P.M. and wakening at 2 A.M.).

- *Shift work sleep syndrome* occurs when patients are required to work during sleep times.

Treatment

- A light box (2,500–10,000 lux) can be used to push sleep initiation later in the evening (advanced sleep phase syndrome) or earlier in the evening (delayed sleep phase syndrome).

- The melatonin agonist ramelteon can be used.

TABLE 6–5. DSM-IV-TR diagnostic criteria for circadian rhythm sleep disorder

---

A. A persistent or recurrent pattern of sleep disruption leading to excessive sleepiness or insomnia that is due to a mismatch between the sleep-wake schedule required by a person's environment and his or her circadian sleep-wake pattern.

B. The sleep disturbance causes clinically significant distress or impairment in social, occupational, or other important areas of functioning.

C. The disturbance does not occur exclusively during the course of another sleep disorder or other mental disorder.

D. The disturbance is not due to the direct physiological effects of a substance (e.g., a drug of abuse, a medication) or a general medical condition.

Specify type:

.31 Delayed sleep phase type: a persistent pattern of late sleep onset and late awakening times, with an inability to fall asleep and awaken at a desired earlier time

.35 Jet lag type: sleepiness and alertness that occur at an inappropriate time of day relative to local time, occurring after repeated travel across more than one time zone

.36 Shift work type: insomnia during the major sleep period or excessive sleepiness during the major awake period associated with night shift work or frequently changing shift work

.30 Unspecified type

Parasomnias

The stages of sleep are non-REM (NREM; further divided into stages 1, 2, 3, and 4) and REM sleep. Parasomnias are disorders of arousal occurring in NREM (stages 2–4) and REM sleep.

NREM Parasomnias

NREM parasomnias occur in the first half of the night, during NREM sleep, and the patient is amnestic for the event.

- *Sleepwalking disorder* (Table 6–6) involves arousal from sleep and the performance of complex motor activity (e.g., dressing, eating, walking). It usually occurs only once each night, not multiple times. If the patient is forced awake, violence is common. Any condition that may cause arousals from NREM sleep may precipitate sleepwalking (e.g., OSA in an obese child). If sleepwalking occurs with adult onset, consider nocturnal seizures rather than sleepwalking as a diagnosis.

- *Sleep terrors disorder* (Table 6–7) presents as an abrupt awakening from sleep usually beginning with a piercing scream and fear with sympathetic response. The patient is confused and disoriented and will have little memory of the event. Patients and their families should be warned that the development of sleep terrors increases the chance of sleepwalking. Sleep terrors occur from NREM, whereas nightmares occur from REM.

- *Confusional arousals* include awakenings with imbalance and psychomotor slowing induced by a forced arousal, frequently by a family member.

ASSESSMENT

Evaluation of NREM parasomnias should focus on conditions that may disrupt sleep (e.g., comorbid OSA, reflux) or may result in rebound of NREM sleep (e.g., sleep deprivation, medication initiation or cessation). If the disorder is resulting in injury to the patient, there is complaint of excessive daytime sleepiness, or there is suspicion of comorbid disorder such as OSA, a polysomnogram is warranted.

TREATMENT

- *Education* about the disorder should be provided to the patient and family members. Family members must be advised to gently guide the patient back to bed during an attack. Any potentially harmful elements (e.g., guns) should be locked up or removed from the house.

- *Medication* should be reserved for patients who are having frequent events or are dangerous to themselves or others. Benzodiazepines are the mainstay of treatment, including diazepam and clonazepam. Selective serotonin reuptake inhibitors (SSRIs) can be used if there is a contraindication to the benzodiazepines.

TABLE 6–6.   DSM-IV-TR criteria for sleepwalking disorder

A.   Repeated episodes of rising from bed during sleep and walking about, usually occurring during the first third of the major sleep episode.

B.   While sleepwalking, the person has a blank, staring face, is relatively unresponsive to the efforts of others to communicate with him or her, and can be awakened only with great difficulty.

C.   On awakening (either from the sleepwalking episode or the next morning), the person has amnesia for the episode.

D.   Within several minutes after awakening from the sleepwalking episode, there is no impairment of mental activity or behavior (although there may initially be a short period of confusion or disorientation).

E.   The sleepwalking causes clinically significant distress or impairment in social, occupational, or other important areas of functioning.

F.   The disturbance is not due to the direct physiological effects of a substance (e.g., a drug of abuse, a medication) or a general medical condition.

TABLE 6–7.   DSM-IV-TR criteria for sleep terror disorder

A.   Recurrent episodes of abrupt awakening from sleep, usually occurring during the first third of the major sleep episode and beginning with a panicky scream.

B.   Intense fear and signs of autonomic arousal, such as tachycardia, rapid breathing, and sweating, during each episode.

C.   Relative unresponsiveness to efforts of others to comfort the person during the episode.

D.   No detailed dream is recalled and there is amnesia for the episode.

E.   The episodes cause clinically significant distress or impairment in social, occupational, or other important areas of functioning.

F.   The disturbance is not due to the direct physiological effects of a substance (e.g., a drug of abuse, a medication) or a general medical condition.

- *Behavioral treatment* for children is appropriate if the terror or behavior occurs at approximately the same time nightly. The child is awoken prior to the anticipated time of event for 4 weeks and allowed to go back to sleep.

REM Parasomnias

REM parasomnias occur in the second half of the night, or are of short duration, and are remembered by the patient.

REM behavior disorder (RBD) occurs from the loss of normal REM sleep atonia (lack of movement), resulting in dream enactment. Patients may punch, kick, run, and injure themselves or a bed partner. This may occur multiple times during the night as REM periods occur.

- Men are more affected by RBD than are women.

- RBD may be induced by medication, including tricyclic antidepressants, monoamine oxidase inhibitors, and SSRIs, or by the withdrawal of alcohol or benzodiazepines.

- Up to 60% of patients with chronic RBD develop Parkinson's disease, multiple system atrophy, or Lewy body dementia (Boeve et al. 2003; Gagnon et al. 2006)

Nightmare disorder (Table 6–8) includes recurrent and distressing dreams that include vivid imagery. Precipitants can be stress, medical infection, or any medications that alter norepinephrine, serotonin, acetylcholine, or γ-aminobutyric acid (common with SSRIs). Treatment consists of changing the offending medication, treating the medical condition, or behavioral treatment.

ASSESSMENT

- History and physical examination should focus on signs or symptoms of neurological disorders listed in the previous section or brainstem pathology (e.g., resting tremor, bradykinesia, dementia, impaired eye movements) and medication additions or changes.

- Polysomnography may not capture an event but will show an increase in the chin electromyelogram (EMG) during REM (normally patients are atonic during REM) and increased electromyographic activity from the limbs. Additional arm EMG leads may be added if RBD is a concern.

TABLE 6–8. DSM-IV-TR criteria for nightmare disorder

A. Repeated awakenings from the major sleep period or naps with detailed recall of extended and extremely frightening dreams, usually involving threats to survival, security, or self-esteem. The awakenings generally occur during the second half of the sleep period.

B. On awakening from the frightening dreams, the person rapidly becomes oriented and alert (in contrast to the confusion and disorientation seen in sleep terror disorder and some forms of epilepsy).

C. The dream experience, or the sleep disturbance resulting from the awakening, causes clinically significant distress or impairment in social, occupational, or other important areas of functioning.

D. The nightmares do not occur exclusively during the course of another mental disorder (e.g., a delirium, posttraumatic stress disorder) and are not due to the direct physiological effects of a substance (e.g., a drug of abuse, a medication) or a general medical condition.

- MRI without contrast is appropriate to exclude structural pathology in the brainstem or midbrain.

TREATMENT

Treatment should be focused on patient and bed partner safety (bed partner should sleep separately until disorder is controlled).

- First-line therapies are clonazepam 0.5–2 mg qhs or temazepam 15–45 mg qhs. The mechanism of action for benzodiazepine treatment is not the suppression of sleep stages 3 and 4 but rather a decreased arousal threshold that prevents patients from waking up and acting out dreams.
- Second-line medications include donepezil 5 mg qhs, ropinirole (Requip; titrate to a maximum of 1mg tid) or pramipexole (Mirapex; 0.125–0.75 mg) at bedtime, and less frequently, tricyclic antidepressants.

References

American Psychiatric Association: Diagnostic and Statistical Manual of Mental Disorders, 4th Edition, Text Revision. Washington, DC, American Psychiatric Association, 2000

Boeve BF, Silber MH, Parisi JE: Synucleinopathy pathology and REM sleep behavior disorder plus dementia or parkinsonism. Neurology 61:40–45, 2003

Buchner NJ, Sanner BM, Borgel J, et al: Continuous positive airway pressure treatment of mild to moderate obstructive sleep apnea reduces cardiovascular risk. Am J Respir Crit Care Med 176:1274–1280, 2007

Gagnon JF, Postuma RB, Mazza S, et al: Rapid-eye-movement sleep behaviour disorder and neurodegenerative diseases. Lancet Neurol 5:424–432, 2006

Marangell LB, Martinez JM: Concise Guide to Psychopharmacology, 2nd Edition. Washington, DC, American Psychiatric Publishing, 2006

Roth T, Seiden D, Sainati S, et al: Effects of ramelteon on patients-reported sleep latency in older adults with chronic insomnia. Sleep Med 7:312–118, 2006a

Roth T, White D, Schmidt-Nowara W: Effects of armodafinil in the treatment of residual excessive sleepiness associated with obstructive sleep apnea/hypopnea syndrome: a 12-week, multicenter, double-blind, randomized, placebo-controlled study in nCPAP-adherent adults. Clin Ther 28:689–706, 2006b

Schechter MS: Technical report: diagnosis and management of childhood obstructive sleep apnea syndrome. Pediatrics 109:e69, 2002

7

Substance-Related Disorders

Substance-related disorders, including both abuse and dependence, are common and devastating diseases. Accurate assessment is critical to the care of every patient undergoing psychiatric evaluation. The prevalence of of substance-related disorders is shown in Table 7–1.

Key Points

- Assessment of substance use must be included in all evaluations.

- Most patients underestimate their substance intake when reporting to physicians.

- It is better to ask "How much do you use X?" than "Do you use X?" or "You don't use X, do you?"

- For each substance used, inquire about

  - Onset, frequency, duration, route, patterns, and circumstances of use;

  - Timing and amount of most recent use; and

  - Degree of intoxication and withdrawal.

- Psychiatric comorbidity is extremely common; it is often useful to try to determine if the substance use started before the other psychiatric disorder (e.g., depression), or if the other psychiatric disorder occurred first and led to subsequent substance abuse.

TABLE 7–1. Prevalence of substance-related disorders

DISORDER	12-MONTH PREVALENCE	LIFETIME PREVALENCE
Alcohol abuse	3.1	13.2
Alcohol dependence	1.3	5.4
Drug abuse	1.4	7.9
Drug dependence	0.4	3.9
Any substance disorder	3.8	14.6

Source. Data from Kessler et al. 2005a, 2005b.

- Alcohol and sedative-hypnotic withdrawal is potentially life-threatening.
- Withdrawal from opiates is extremely uncomfortable.
- Substances that do not induce physical tolerance, and therefore lead to minimal withdrawal, include marijuana and hallucinogens.
- Alcoholics Anonymous (AA), Narcotics Anonymous (NA), and other 12-step programs are often vital to recovery. The Web sites of these organizations list services in the patient's geographical area (see, e.g., www.alcoholics-anonymous.org and www.na.org).
- Pharmacotherapy, when available for the treatment of a specific substance use disorder, is rarely appropriate as monotherapy.

General Concepts and Definitions

- *Intoxication.* The acute effects of overdosage of chemical substances. Characteristically, intoxication with substances of abuse produces behavioral or psychological changes because of their effects on the central nervous system. Such changes may be expressed as belligerence, differences in mood, or impaired judgment. The DSM-IV-TR diagnostic criteria for substance intoxication are presented in Table 7–2 (American Psychiatric Association 2000).
- *Abuse.* Impairment in social and occupational functioning resulting from the pathological and "compulsive" use of a substance. The concept is closely related to the definition of substance dependence, which has similar symptoms of impairment but may include evidence of physiological tolerance or withdrawal. Typi-

---

TABLE 7–2. DSM-IV-TR criteria for substance intoxication

A. The development of a reversible substance-specific syndrome due to recent ingestion of (or exposure to) a substance. **Note:** Different substances may produce similar or identical syndromes.

B. Clinically significant maladaptive behavioral or psychological changes that are due to the effect of the substance on the central nervous system (e.g., belligerence, mood lability, cognitive impairment, impaired judgment, impaired social or occupational functioning) and develop during or shortly after use of the substance.

C. The symptoms are not due to a general medical condition and are not better accounted for by another mental disorder.

---

cal symptoms of abuse include failure to fulfill major role obligations at work, school, or home; recurrent use of the substance in situations in which such use is physically hazardous; substance-related legal problems; and continued use even though it causes or exaggerates interpersonal problems. The DSM-IV-TR diagnostic criteria for substance abuse are presented in Table 7–3.

- *Dependence.*   Chemical dependence; sometimes defined in terms of physiological dependence, as evidenced by tolerance or withdrawal; at other times, defined in terms of impairment in social and occupational functioning resulting from the pathological and repeated use of a substance. In the latter definition, tolerance and withdrawal symptoms may be present but are not essential. The DSM-IV-TR diagnostic criteria for substance dependence are presented in Table 7–4.

- *Withdrawal.*   The constellation of symptoms and signs that develops within a short period (usually hours) after cessation or significant reduction of use of a substance in a person with a pattern of heavy or prolonged use of that substance. The withdrawal symptoms tend to be specific for each substance. The DSM-IV-TR diagnostic criteria for substance intoxication are presented in Table 7–5.

- *Substance-induced psychiatric disorders.*   Mental syndromes secondary to the use of drugs (including alcohol). In DSM-IV-TR, these disorders (except for intoxication and withdrawal) are placed in the diagnostic categories with which they share phenomenology. For example, substance-induced mood disorder is listed under mood disorders, and substance-induced sleep disor-

---

TABLE 7–3.   **DSM-IV-TR criteria for substance abuse**

A.   A maladaptive pattern of substance use leading to clinically significant impairment or distress, as manifested by one (or more) of the following, occurring within a 12-month period:

  (1)   recurrent substance use resulting in a failure to fulfill major role obligations at work, school, or home (e.g., repeated absences or poor work performance related to substance use; substance-related absences, suspensions, or expulsions from school; neglect of children or household)

  (2)   recurrent substance use in situations in which it is physically hazardous (e.g., driving an automobile or operating a machine when impaired by substance use)

  (3)   recurrent substance-related legal problems (e.g., arrests for substance-related disorderly conduct)

  (4)   continued substance use despite having persistent or recurrent social or interpersonal problems caused or exacerbated by the effects of the substance (e.g., arguments with spouse about consequences of intoxication, physical fights)

B.   The symptoms have never met the criteria for substance dependence for this class of substance.

---

der is listed under sleep disorders. The relevant diagnostic categories are delirium, dementia, amnestic disorder, psychotic disorder (with delusions or hallucinations), mood disorder, anxiety disorder, sleep disorder, and sexual dysfunction.

General Treatment Principles

- Substance use disorders include both psychological and physiological components.

- Pharmacotherapies are useful and sometimes necessary to treat withdrawal and often increase the chance of success for longer-term abstinence. However, substance use disorders also include complex social and psychological components that cannot be ignored.

- Education about the impact of substances on the patient's life and about social circumstances that may trigger relapse, as well as learning new coping mechanisms, are key components of treatment.

TABLE 7–4. **DSM-IV-TR criteria for substance dependence**

A maladaptive pattern of substance use, leading to clinically significant impairment or distress, as manifested by three (or more) of the following, occurring at any time in the same 12-month period:

(1) tolerance, as defined by either of the following:

   (a) a need for markedly increased amounts of the substance to achieve intoxication or desired effect

   (b) markedly diminished effect with continued use of the same amount of the substance

(2) withdrawal, as manifested by either of the following:

   (a) the characteristic withdrawal syndrome for the substance (refer to criteria A and B of the criteria sets for withdrawal from the specific substances)

   (b) the same (or a closely related) substance is taken to relieve or avoid withdrawal symptoms

(3) the substance is often taken in larger amounts or over a longer period than was intended

(4) there is a persistent desire or unsuccessful efforts to cut down or control substance use

(5) a great deal of time is spent in activities necessary to obtain the substance (e.g., visiting multiple doctors or driving long distances), use the substance (e.g., chain-smoking), or recover from its effects

(6) important social, occupational, or recreational activities are given up or reduced because of substance use

(7) the substance use is continued despite knowledge of having a persistent or recurrent physical or psychological problem that is likely to have been caused or exacerbated by the substance (e.g., current cocaine use despite recognition of cocaine-induced depression, or continued drinking despite recognition that an ulcer was made worse by alcohol consumption)

TABLE 7–4.   DSM-IV-TR criteria for substance dependence (*continued*)

Specify if:

With physiological dependence: evidence of tolerance or withdrawal (i.e., either Item 1 or 2 is present)

Without physiological dependence: no evidence of tolerance or withdrawal (i.e., neither Item 1 nor 2 is present)

Course specifiers:

Early full remission: For at least 1 month but less than 12 months, no criteria for dependence or abuse have been met.

Early partial remission: For at least 1 month but less than 12 months, one or more criteria have been met (but the full criteria are not met).

Sustained full remission: None of the criteria for dependence or abuse have been met for 12 months or longer.

Sustained partial remission: Full criteria for dependence have not been met for a period of 12 months or longer; however, one or more criteria for dependence or abuse have been met.

On agonist therapy: An individual is on a prescribed agonist (e.g., methadone) and no criteria have been met for at least the past month (except tolerance to or withdrawal from the agonist).

In a controlled environment: An individual is in a setting that restricts access to substances (e.g., jail or a locked hospital unit) and no criteria have been met for at least 1 month.

TABLE 7–5.   DSM-IV-TR criteria for substance withdrawal

A. The development of a substance-specific syndrome due to the cessation of (or reduction in) substance use that has been heavy and prolonged.

B. The substance-specific syndrome causes clinically significant distress or impairment in social, occupational, or other important areas of functioning.

C. The symptoms are not due to a general medical condition and are not better accounted for by another mental disorder.

Alcohol Dependence

- Alcohol dependence can result in gastrointestinal, hematological, endocrinological, neurological, and cardiovascular problems (Table 7–6).
- Withdrawal symptoms may be seen with decreased intake, even if some intake continues.
- Withdrawal may include seizures, peaking 24 hours after the last drink.
- Delirium tremens (DTs) may include autonomic instability and hallucinations. DTs typically occur 2–3 days after significant decrease in alcohol consumption and peak at days 4–5.
- Wernicke's encephalopathy is a disease due to a nutritional deficiency of vitamin B_1 (thiamine), which provokes acute mental confusion, ataxia, and ophthalmoplegia (paralysis of some or all muscles of the eye).
- Korsakoff syndrome (alcohol amnestic disorder) is a disease associated with chronic alcoholism (alcohol dependence) and result-

TABLE 7–6. **Associated medical complications of alcohol dependence**

Gastrointestinal	Fatty liver deposits, hepatitis, cirrhosis, pancreatitis, gastric bleeding, hepatic dysregulation
Hematological	Anemia; impaired immune functioning; increased oropharyngeal, esophageal, gastric, hepatic, and pancreatic cancer
Endocrinological	In men: testicular atrophy, decreased testosterone levels, body hair loss, and gynecomastia secondary to increased estrogen levels
	In women: infertility, reduced menstruation, changes in secondary sex characteristics secondary to gonadal failure
Neurological	Increased risk of cerebrovascular accident, cerebellar degeneration (slow process), peripheral neuropathy, dementia
Cardiovascular	Increased blood pressure, cardiomyopathy, heart failure

ing from a deficiency of vitamin B_1. Patients sustain damage to part of the thalamus and cerebellum and have anterograde and retrograde amnesia, with an inability to retain new information. Other symptoms include inflammation of nerves, muttering delirium, insomnia, illusions, and hallucinations. In alcohol amnestic disorder, unlike dementia, other intellectual functions may be preserved.

- Large amounts of alcohol, particularly if consumed rapidly, can produce partial (i.e., fragmentary) or complete (i.e., en bloc) blackouts, which are periods of memory loss for events that transpired while a person was drinking.

Risk Factors

About 50% of the risk of alcohol dependence is genetic. Environmental risk factors, which predominate in adolescence, include childhood abuse and trauma, family influences, peer relationships, and stress (Hasin et al. 2007).

Subtypes

- **Type I alcoholism:** Heavy use generally begins after age 25 and is reinforced by external circumstances. The person is able to abstain for long periods and frequently feels guilt, fear, and loss of control regarding alcohol dependency.
- **Type II alcoholism:** Onset is generally before age 25, and there is more spontaneous alcohol seeking regardless of external circumstances. Fights and arrests are common, and the person rarely feels guilt about alcohol dependency.

Screening

CAGE is a brief questionnaire that is useful in screening for alcoholism:
C   Have you ever tried to cut down on your intake?
A   Have you ever been annoyed by criticism of your drinking?
G   Have you ever felt guilty about your drinking?
E   Do you ever have an eye-opener (drinking in the morning to treat a hangover)?

Useful laboratory markers are listed in Table 7–7.

TABLE 7–7. Laboratory markers of heavy drinking

MARKER	MEN (VALUE SUGGESTING HEAVY DRINKING)	WOMEN (VALUE SUGGESTING HEAVY DRINKING)	ACCURACY
Carbohydrate-deficient transferrin (CDT)	>20 U/L	>26 U/L	Very good
γ-Glutamyltransferase (GGT)	>35 U/L	>30 U/L	Very good
Mean corpuscular volume (MCV)	>91 μm³	>91 μm³	Good
Aspartate aminotransferase (AST)	>40 U/L	>33 U/L	Fair
Alanine aminotransferase (ALT)	>46 U/L	>35 U/L	Fair
Uric acid	>8.0 mg/dL	>6.2 mg/dL	Fair
5-Hydroxytryptophol-to-hydroxyindoleacetic acid ratio	>20	>20	Fair

Source. Data from Schuckit and Tapert 2004.

Outpatient Treatment for Alcohol Dependence

Patients with alcohol dependence may be treated in an outpatient setting if their clinical condition and environmental and social circumstances do not require a higher level of inpatient care. The American Psychiatric Association (2006) Practice Guidelines list absolute contraindications and relative contraindications to outpatient treatment.

ABSOLUTE CONTRAINDICATIONS

- Coexisting acute or chronic illness (e.g., severe cardiac disease)
- Delirium
- No reliable person to help monitor patient out of hospital
- Pregnancy
- Seizure disorder or prior seizures in withdrawal
- Suicide risk

RELATIVE CONTRAINDICATIONS

- History of previous unsuccessful outpatient detoxification
- Comorbid benzodiazepine dependence
- High risk of severe withdrawal
  - Age >40 years
  - Heavy drinking for >8 years
  - Drinking greater than 1 pint of alcohol or eight 12-oz beers daily
  - Cirrhosis
  - Increased mean corpuscular volume
  - Increased blood urea nitrogen

Treatment of Alcohol Withdrawal Syndrome (Detoxification)

- Identify and treat comorbid medical problems.
- Ensure adequate fluids and electrolytes.

- Prescribe B vitamins. Alcohol interferes with the absorption of these vitamins, which are not well stored and are needed to prevent and treat alcohol-related neurological disturbances.
  - Prescribe thiamine 100 mg/day po or im and then 50 mg/month.
  - Prescribe folate 1 mg/day or a multivitamin daily.

- Longer-acting benzodiazepines, such as chlordiazepoxide (Librium) or diazepam (Valium), are often preferred to suppress symptoms of acute alcohol withdrawal because these medications in essence self-taper. For example, prescribe chlordiazepoxide 25–50 mg po up to 4 times/day unless patient is sleepy or light-headed; taper by 25% per day.

- If hepatic function is impaired, oxazepam (Serax) is preferred because it is not hepatically metabolized.

Pharmacological Prevention of Relapse

NALTREXONE (REVIA)

- Mechanism: Naltrexone is an opioid antagonist that is also thought to be a μ opioid partial agonist. It normalizes β-endorphin levels, which are decreased in some abstinent alcoholics. As such, it decreases craving. Because of the antagonist activity, endorphin levels do not rise after alcohol intake, which inhibits the reinforcing effect of an initial drink after a period of sobriety.
- Dosage: 50 mg po daily
- Key side effects: nausea, vomiting, abdominal pain, constipation, nervousness, headache, insomnia, sedation

ACAMPROSATE (CAMPRAL)

- Mechanism: modulates glutamate/N-methyl-D-aspartate (NMDA) activity; γ-aminobutyric acid (GABA) agonist
- Dosage: 666 mg tid
- Key side effect: diarrhea

DISULFIRAM (ANTABUSE)

- Mechanism: Acetaldehyde is the first metabolic product of ethanol. Disulfiram inhibits the enzyme acetaldehyde dehydrogenase, which leads to the accumulation of acetaldehyde, resulting in flushing, sweating, and tachycardia. If more alcohol is consumed, dyspnea, nausea, and vomiting may also occur.

- Dosage: 250–500 mg/day
- Key side effect: fatigue
- Possible side effect: hepatotoxicity
- Disulfiram is an irreversible enzyme inhibitor, so reaction to alcohol may occur up to 2 weeks after stopping the medication while new enzyme is synthesized in the absence of the drug. *Advise patients to avoid alcohol in all forms, including foods and over-the-counter (OTC) medications.*

Sedatives and Hypnotics

- Sedative-hypnotic intoxication and withdrawal are similar to alcohol intoxication and withdrawal.
- Sedative-hypnotic withdrawal is life-threatening.
- Barbiturates, benzodiazepines, and alcohol exhibit cross-tolerance, defined as the extension of tolerance to a substance developed over a period of long-term administration to another substance to which an individual has not been previously exposed. A person who has developed tolerance to alcohol will have a diminished response to the usual dose of a benzodiazepine because tolerance to alcohol has induced tolerance to the benzodiazepine's effect.
- Alprazolam can be tapered by decreasing the dose 0.25 mg/week.
- Overdose is lethal with barbiturates. The effects of benzodiazepines are mediated by endogenous GABA; as such, uncomplicated benzodiazepine overdoses are often not lethal unless combined with alcohol or barbiturates.
- Benzodiazepines when used in patients without substance abuse and without self-escalation rarely result in abuse, although there may be physiological dependence.
- The goal of barbiturate detoxification is to prevent the occurrence of major symptoms and to minimize the development of intolerable symptoms. The regimen must be individualized, but the initial reduction is typically 10% of the daily stabilization dose (Ciraulo et al. 2005). Table 7–8 presents guidelines for barbiturate detoxification using the pentobarbital tolerance test.

TABLE 7–8. Guidelines for barbiturate detoxification

SYMPTOMS AFTER TEST DOSE OF 200 MG OF ORAL PENTOBARBITAL	ESTIMATED 24-HOUR ORAL PENTOBARBITAL DOSE (MG)	ESTIMATED 24-HOUR ORAL PHENOBARBITAL DOSE (MG)
Asleep, but can be aroused	0	0
Sedated, drowsy, slurred speech, nystagmus, ataxia, positive Romberg test result	500–600	150–200
Few signs of intoxication, patient is comfortable, may have lateral nystagmus	800	250
No drug effect	1,000–1,200	300–400

Note. Maximum phenobarbital dose is 600 mg.
Source. Adapted from Ciraulo et al. 2005.

Opioids

Opioids include heroin, morphine, methadone, and other prescription narcotics.

- Intoxication symptoms include analgesia, sedation, euphoria, and apathy.
- Withdrawal peaks in 2–3 days and resolves in 2 weeks; it is not life-threatening. Symptoms include anxiety, sweating, rhinorrhea, dilated pupils, chills, muscle cramps, and increased blood pressure and heart rate.
- Complications of opioid use include decreased gastric motility, lymphadenopathy, vein sclerosis, edema, and ulceration.
  - With intravenous administration, complications include bacterial infection, emboli, HIV, hepatitis, endocarditis, meningitis, brain abscess, and septicemia.
  - Overdose results in death from respiratory depression.

Pharmacological Treatment

BUPRENORPHINE

- Lower overdose potential and abuse liability than opioids of abuse
- Less severe withdrawal than methadone when discontinued (Kosten and Kleber 1988)
- Comparable to methadone in treatment retention and reduced heroin abuse
- Mechanism: partial opioid agonist
- Maintenance dosage: 8–32 mg/day sl
- Common side effect: euphoria

SUBOXONE (BUPRENORPHINE/NALOXONE)

- Combination has less abuse potential than buprenorphine alone, because the naloxone blocks the euphoric effect.
- Suboxone can precipitate withdrawal.
- Table 7–9 presents dosing guidelines.

TABLE 7–9. Buprenorphine/naloxone induction schedule

PATIENT TYPE	DAY 1		DAY 2
	FIRST DOSE	SUPPLEMENTAL DOSE	
Not currently dependent	2/0.5 mg		4/1 mg
Dependent on heroin or pain medications	2/0.5 to 4/1 mg[a]	Redose every 1–2 hours; if withdrawal continues, up to a total of 8/2 mg.	If the patient is still in withdrawal, give first-day dose plus 2/0.5 to 4/1 mg.
Dependent on methadone (≤30 mg/day) or on LAAM (≤40 mg/every other day)[b]	2/0.5 mg[a]	Redose every 1–2 hours; if withdrawal continues, up to a total of 8/2 mg.	If the patient is still in withdrawal, give first-day dose plus 2/0.5 to 4/1 mg; if oversedated, give <8/2 mg.

Note.   LAAM=L-α-acetylmethadol (no longer available in the United States). Buprenorphine/naloxone tablets are administered sublingually; dose amounts consist of the buprenorphine dose (the number before the slash) and the naloxone dose (the number after the slash).

[a]Do not begin buprenorphine until patient shows evidence of opioid withdrawal.
[b]Patient should abstain from LAAM for ≥48 hours before first buprenorphine dose.
Source.   Adapted from Epstein et al. 2005.

CLONIDINE (CATAPRES)

- Mechanism: Clonidine is an α_2-adrenergic agonist that suppresses opiate withdrawal.
- Dosing: Prescribe a test dose of 0.1 mg followed by 0.1–0.4 mg every 4–6 hours for 6 days, then taper over 4 days.
- Clonidine should be used only if the clinician is experienced with the method.
- Common side effects: hypotension, sedation, dry mouth

METHADONE MAINTENANCE

- High doses alleviate craving and induce cross-tolerance to other opioids.
- Common side effects: euphoria, drowsiness

Hallucinogens

Table 7–10 lists hallucinogens and their street names.

- Intoxication symptoms include altered perception, hallucinations (especially visual), illusions, derealization, and anxiety.
- Treatment of intoxication consists of maintaining a calm environment and the as-needed use of benzodiazepines and occasionally antipsychotics, if the psychotic features are severe. This is most common with phencyclidine (PCP), where patients may become violent.
- Withdrawal is not common. Longer-term treatment consists of education and 12-step programs.

Stimulants

Stimulants include amphetamines and cocaine. The smoked form of stimulants is more potent and addictive than oral or intranasal administration. Smoked cocaine is called "crack;" smoked amphetamine is called "ice."

- There is no true withdrawal with stimulants, but chronic daily users may report fatigue, depression, and hypersomnolence.

TABLE 7–10. Street names of hallucinogens

HALLUCINOGEN	STREET NAME
LSD (lysergic acid diethylamide)	Acid, blotter, blue devils, California sunshine, haze, microdot, mickey, Mr. Natural, paper acid, purple haze, sunshine, wedges, window pane
Morning glory seeds	Flying saucers, licorice drops, heavenly gates, pearly gates
PCP (phencyclidine)	Angel dust
Psilocybin	Magic mushrooms, mushroom
DMT (*N,N*-dimethyltryptamine), DET (*N,N*-diethyltryptamine)	Businessman's lunch, snuff
Peyote/mescaline	Button(s), cactus, mesc, mescal, mescal buttons, moon, peyote
DOM (2,5-dimethoxy-4-methyl-amphetamine)	Golden eagle, STP, psychodrine, title
MDA (3,4-methylenedioxy-amphetamine)	Love drug
MDMA (3,4-methylenedioxy-methamphetamine)	Adam, Ecstasy, MDM, XTC
MDEA (3,4-methylenedioxy-ethyl-amphetamine)	Eve

Source. Adapted from Tacke and Ebert 2005.

- Multiple pharmacological agents have been used to reduce relapse (e.g., desipramine, bromocriptine, naltrexone), but none are a standard of care.
- Treatment consists of education and 12-step programs.

Club Drugs

γ-Hydroxybutyric Acid (GHB)

A metabolite of GABA, GHB is approved by the U.S. Food and Drug Administration for the treatment of the cataplexy of narcolepsy.

- Intoxication symptoms include sedation, euphoria, and sexual disinhibition.

- Withdrawal is similar to barbiturate withdrawal.

- Pharmacological treatment of withdrawal is with benzodiazepines. High dosages may be required, up to 10 mg lorazepam intravenously per hour (Craig et al. 2000). The phenobarbital protocol may also be used. Some patients will require antipsychotics, but these medications are a last resort because patients in GHB withdrawal are often hyperpyrexic, which may increase the risk of neuroleptic malignant syndrome.

- Longer-term treatment involves drug counseling and 12-step programs.

Ecstasy

Ecstasy (3,4-methylenedioxymethamphetamine [MDMA]) is chemically similar to both amphetamines and mescaline.

- Intoxication symptoms include increased energy, increased mental clarity, and a feeling of closeness to others and well-being. Rebound depression and anxiety may occur the next day.

- The drug appears to transiently lessen normal psychological defenses, which is part of its appeal as a drug of abuse and also why some therapists have advocated the judicious use of Ecstasy as part of psychotherapy.

- Some data suggest that use of Ecstasy may permanently destroy serotonin neurons (McCann et al. 2000). Longer-term effects of memory impairment and cognition have been reported with chronic use.

- Treatment is the same as for amphetamine abuse.

Cannabis

- Intoxication symptoms include euphoria, increased appetite, dry mouth, anxiety, impaired coordination, and sedation. Chronic use is associated with decreased motivation.

- Treatment involves drug counseling and 12-step programs.

- Pharmacotherapy is typically not needed. There is no true withdrawal, but chronic users may describe irritability and insomnia when stopping daily use.

Nicotine

Nicotine replacement results in approximately twice the successful quit rate of treatment without replacement. All types of nicotine replacement should be combined with behavioral interventions, and the replacement should be tapered over 2–3 months.

- Nicotine gum is available OTC in 2-mg and 4-mg strengths. Instruct the patient to chew a few times and then park the gum on the side of the inner mouth to avoid exposure to too much nicotine at once.
- Nicotine lozenges are available OTC in 2-mg and 4-mg strengths. A nicotine lozenge releases 25% more nicotine per milligram compared with nicotine gum. The lozenge contains phenylalanine.
- Transdermal nicotine is available in a variety of formulations OTC. The typical program is an 8-week taper. There is less abuse potential with transdermal nicotine than with as-needed nicotine replacement.
- A nicotine nasal inhaler is available by prescription. It offers the most rapid delivery of nicotine, compared with other nicotine replacement products.
- A nicotine oral inhaler is available by prescription. It mimics the ritual of smoking more than other products. It should be tapered over 3–6 months. The nicotine oral inhaler is relatively contraindicated in patients with asthma.

Non-nicotine pharmacotherapies include bupropion SR (Zyban):

- 150 mg po for 4 days, then 150 mg bid; smoking is ceased on day 8.

Varenicline (Chantix) is started one week before the intended date to stop smoking. The manufacturer recommends that the medication be taken after eating and with a full glass of water. Dosing titration is as follows:

- Days 1–3: 0.5 mg qd
- Days 4–7: 0.5 mg bid
- Day 8 through end of treatment: 1 mg bid

For patients who successfully quit with 12 weeks of treatment, an additional 12 weeks of treatment is recommended. Due to the mechanism of action, patients taking varenicline should not use nicotine substitution products designed to assist in smoking cessation. The most common side effects are dose dependent nausea, insomnia, and gastrointestinal distress. Varenicline has been associated with changes in behavior, agitation, depressed mood, and suicidal thoughts and actions. Preexisting psychiatric illness may worsen and patients should be carefully observed for new or worsening psychiatric symptoms.

References

American Psychiatric Association: Diagnostic and Statistical Manual of Mental Disorders, 4th Edition, Text Revision. Washington, DC, American Psychiatric Association, 2000

American Psychiatric Association: Quick Reference to the American Psychiatric Association Practice Guidelines for the Treatment of Psychiatric Disorders, Compendium 2006. Washington, DC, American Psychiatric Publishing, 2006

Ciraulo DA, Ciraulo JA, Sands BF, et al: Sedative-hypnotics, in Clinical Manual of Addiction Psychopharmacology. Edited by Kranzler HR, Ciraulo DA. Washington, DC, American Psychiatric Publishing, 2005, pp 111–162

Craig K, Gomez HF, McManus JL, et al: Severe gamma-hydroxybutyrate withdrawal: a case report and literature review. J Emerg Med 18:65–70, 2000

Epstein S, Renner JA Jr, Ciraulo AD, et al: Opioids, in Clinical Manual of Addiction Psychopharmacology. Edited by Kranzler HR, Ciraulo DA. Washington, DC, American Psychiatric Publishing, 2005, pp 55–110

Hasin D, Hatzenbuehler ML, Keyes-Wild K, et al: Vulnerability to alcohol and drug use disorders, in Recognition and Prevention of Major Mental and Substance Use Disorders. Edited by Tsuang MT, Stone WS, Lyons MJ. Washington, DC, American Psychiatric Publishing, 2007, pp 115–155

Kessler RC, Berglund P, Demler O, et al: Lifetime prevalence and age-of-onset distributions of DSM-IV disorders in the National Comorbidity Survey Replication. Arch Gen Psychiatry 62:593–602, 2005a

Kessler RC, Chiu WT, Demler O, et al: Prevalence, severity, and comorbidity of 12-month DSM-IV disorders in the National Comorbidity Survey Replication. Arch Gen Psychiatry 62:617–627, 2005b

Kosten TR, Kleber HD: Buprenorphine detoxification from opioid dependence: a pilot study. Life Sci 42:635–641, 1988

McCann UD, Eligulashvili V, Ricaurte GA: (+/−)3,4-Methylenedioxymethamphetamine ("Ecstasy")-induced serotonin neurotoxicity: clinical studies. Neuropsychobiology 42:11–16, 2000

Schuckit MA, Tapert S: Alcohol, in The American Psychiatric Publishing Textbook of Substance Abuse Treatment, 3rd Edition. Edited by Galanter M, Kleber HD. Washington, DC, American Psychiatric Publishing, 2004, pp 151–166

Tacke U, Ebert MH: Hallucinogens and phencyclidine, in Clinical Manual of Addiction Psychopharmacology. Edited by Kranzler HR, Ciraulo DA. Washington, DC, American Psychiatric Publishing, 2005, pp 211–241

8

Dementia

Dementia is a syndrome with numerous causes, both reversible or irreversible, and is characterized by impairment in at least three of the following areas: language, memory, visuospatial skills, executive abilities, and emotion. Table 8–1 lists diagnostic features common to all dementias. The most common cause of dementia is Alzheimer's disease. The most important goal in the evaluation of dementia is to look for reversible causes (Table 8–2). Table 8–3 lists the elements of a standard assessment of the dementia patient.

Dementia Subtypes

The dementia subtypes include dementia of the Alzheimer's type, vascular dementia (multi-infarct dementia), dementia due to Pick's disease, dementia due to Creutzfeldt-Jakob disease (also called spongiform encephalopathy), dementia due to HIV disease, dementia due to Parkinson's disease, dementia due to Huntington's disease, dementia due to multiple sclerosis, and substance-induced persisting dementia (Bourgeois et al. 2003).

Dementia of the Alzheimer's Type

- Gradual onset and continuing cognitive decline
- Deficits are not due to other central nervous system, systemic, or substance-induced conditions.
- Manifests most often in seventh and eighth decades

TABLE 8–1. Diagnostic features common to all dementias

Memory impairment	Impaired ability to learn new material or difficulty remembering previously learned material or both (e.g., losing wallet or keys, forgetting food cooking on the stove, getting lost in familiar neighborhood)
Aphasia	Deterioration of language functioning (e.g., difficulty producing names of individuals and objects, use of long and empty phrases, decreased comprehension of spoken and written language). In advanced stages patient may be mute or may speak with echolalia (i.e., repeating what is heard) or palilalia (i.e., repeating sounds or words over and over).
Apraxia	Impaired ability to execute motor activities despite intact motor abilities, sensory function, and comprehension of the required task. Assessment: Ask patient to demonstrate how to brush teeth, arrange sticks in a specific design, etc.
Agnosia	Failure to recognize or identify objects despite intact sensory function. Assessment: Ask patient to identify a key in the hand with eyes closed.
Disturbed executive functioning (especially in disorders of the frontal lobe or associated subcortical pathways)	Executive functioning involves the ability to think abstractly and to plan, initiate, sequence, monitor, and stop complex behavior. Assessment: Ask patient to name as many animals as possible in 1 minute; ask informant about ability to work a planned multistep activity.

Symptoms must be severe enough to cause significant impairment in social or occupational functioning and must represent a decline from previous level of functioning.

Note.   Dementia is not diagnosed if symptoms occur exclusively during the course of delirium. However, if delirium occurs with a preexisting dementia, then both diagnoses are given.
Source.   Adapted from American Psychiatric Association 2000.

TABLE 8–2.   Potentially reversible causes of dementia

Psychiatric	Depression
	Schizophrenia
	Ganser's syndrome (type of factitious disorder in which a patient mimics symptoms associated with dementia and psychosis)
	Malingering
Toxic	Drugs (prescription or street)
	Alcohol
	Chemical poisoning (arsenic, mercury, lead, lithium, and other metals; organic compounds and solvents)
Metabolic	Azotemia/renal failure (diuretics, dehydration, obstruction, hypokalemia)
	Hyponatremia (diuretics, excess antidiuretic hormone, salt wasting, water intoxication)
	Volume depletion
	Hypoglycemia or hyperglycemia
	Hepatic encephalopathy
	Hypothyroidism or hyperthyroidism
	Hyperparathyroidism
	Cushing's syndrome
	Wilson's disease
	Acute intermittent porphyria
Vitamin deficiencies	B_{12}, folic acid, thiamine, niacin
CNS disorders	Vascular (ischemic or hemorrhagic stroke, ischemic-hypoxic brain lesions)
	Trauma (subdural hematoma, postconcussion syndrome)
	Human immunodeficiency virus and opportunistic infections
	Other infections (neurosyphilis, chronic meningitis, brain abscess, progressive multifocal leukoencephalopathy)

TABLE 8–2.	Potentially reversible causes of dementia *(continued)*
CNS disorders *(continued)*	Neoplasm (primary or metastatic)
	Cerebral vasculitis
	Normal-pressure hydrocephalus
	Multiple sclerosis

Source. Adapted from Lipton and Weiner 2003.

- Neuropathology includes neurofibrillary tangles (NFTs), neuritic plaques, and β-amyloid deposits and cerebrocortical atrophy, which predominantly involves the association regions and particularly the medial aspect of the temporal lobe. Although NFTs and plaques are characteristic of dementia of the Alzheimer's type, they are also seen in progressive supranuclear palsy and normal aging, although with different densities and distributions.
- Sundowning (symptoms worsening in the evening)
- Patients with Down syndrome (trisomy 21) are at high risk for developing Alzheimer's disease in middle age.

Vascular Dementia (Multi-Infarct Dementia)

- Second most common dementia
- Focal neurological signs and symptoms or laboratory/radiological evidence indicative of cerebrovascular disease etiologically related to deficits

Dementia Due to Pick's Disease

- Prominent personality changes, especially disinhibition, with relatively spared memory and visuospatial functions
- Age at onset typically 40–60 years
- Executive dysfunction and attentional deficits

Dementia Due to Creutzfeldt-Jakob Disease

- Prion-mediated infection
- Manifests as rapidly progressive cortical dementia accompanied by myoclonus and psychosis

---

TABLE 8–3. Standard assessment of the dementia patient

Laboratory tests

    Complete blood count

    Electrolytes, blood glucose, blood urea nitrogen level

    Thyroid-stimulating hormone level

    Serum vitamin B_{12} level

Neuroimaging

    Computed tomography or magnetic resonance imaging

Systemic assessments

    Electrocardiogram

    Chest X ray

    Urinalysis

    Liver function tests

Optional tests (based on symptoms and examination)

    Lumbar puncture

    Electroencephalogram (EEG) and quantitative EEG

    Single photon emission computed tomography

    Positron emission tomography

    Serum antiphospholipid antibodies

    Serum or urine drug tests

    Serum human immunodeficiency virus antibodies

    Muscle biopsy

    Nerve conduction studies

Source. Adapted from Cummings and Trimble 2002.

Dementia Due to HIV Disease

- Initial symptoms: decreased psychomotor and information processing speed, verbal memory, learning efficiency, and fine motor function

- Later symptoms: decreased executive function, aphasia, apraxia, and agnosia

- Occurs in up to 30% of HIV-positive patients
- Results from neurotoxicity mediated by HIV-infected macrophages

Dementia Due to Parkinson's Disease

- Occurs in 60% of patients with Parkinson's disease
- Symptoms: bradyphrenia, apathy, poor retrieval memory, decreased verbal fluency, and attention deficits

Dementia Due to Huntington's Disease

- Symptoms: impairments in retrieval memory, cognitive speed, concentration, verbal learning, and cognitive flexibility
- High risk for personality change, irritability, aggressive behavior, and suicide

Dementia Due to Multiple Sclerosis

- Occurs in 65% of multiple sclerosis patients
- Symptoms: deficits in memory, attention, information-processing speed, learning, and executive functions
- Language and verbal intelligence are relatively spared.

Substance-Induced Persisting Dementia

- Deficits persist beyond usual duration of substance intoxication or withdrawal, with clinical evidence that deficits are etiologically related to the persisting effects of substance abuse.
- Distinguishing characteristics of cortical and subcortical dementias are shown in Table 8–4.

Differential Diagnosis—Nondementias

- *Mental retardation.*   Onset is before age 18 years (age at onset of dementia is usually late in life). If the onset of the dementia is before age 18 years, both dementia and mental retardation may be diagnosed if the criteria for both disorders are met.
- *Schizophrenia.*   This disorder typically presents in the teens and early twenties with a symptom pattern that includes prominent psychotic symptoms.

TABLE 8–4. Distinguishing characteristics of cortical and subcortical dementias

FUNCTION	CORTICAL DEMENTIA	SUBCORTICAL DEMENTIA
Psychomotor speed	Normal	Slowed
Language	Involved	Spared
Memory		
Recall	Impaired	Impaired
Recognition	Impaired	Spared
Remote	Temporal gradient present	Temporal gradient absent
Executive function	Less involved	More involved
Depression	Less common	More common
Motor system	Spared until late	Involved early
Anatomy	Cerebral cortex	Subcortical structures and dorsolateral prefrontal cortex projecting to head of caudate nucleus
Examples	Alzheimer's disease	Huntington's disease, HIV encephalopathy, lacunar stroke

Note. HIV=human immunodeficiency virus.
Source. Adapted from Cummings and Trimble 2002.

- *Major depressive disorder.* The premorbid state may help to differentiate "pseudodementia" (i.e., cognitive impairments due to the major depressive episode) from dementia. In dementia, there is usually a premorbid history of declining cognitive function, whereas the individual with a major depressive episode is much more likely to have a relatively normal premorbid state and abrupt cognitive decline, with the onset of other symptoms of major depression.

- *Malingering and factitious disorder.* Patterns of cognitive deficits are usually not consistent over time and are not characteristic of those typically seen in dementia (e.g., person may perform calculations while keeping score during a card game but then claim to be unable to perform similar calculations during a mental status examination).

- *Normal decline in cognitive functioning that occurs with aging (as in age-related cognitive decline).*   The diagnosis of dementia is warranted only if there is demonstrable evidence of greater memory and other cognitive impairment than would be expected due to normal aging processes and the symptoms cause impairment in social or occupational functioning.

Treatment

Dementia due to some conditions, such as Alzheimer's disease, can be slowed in the early-to-intermediate stages with medication. Cholinesterase inhibitors are the most widely used (e.g., donepezil, galantamine, rivastigmine; see Chapter 14 of this volume, "Pharmacotherapy"). Memantine may provide cognitive improvement in patients with moderate to severe dementia and can be used in combination with a cholinesterase inhibitor (American Psychiatric Association 2006). Table 8–5 provides pharmacotherapy dosing guidelines for dementia.

- Comorbid depression is common with dementia, and treatment of depression may partially relieve symptoms of dementia.
- Treat underlying conditions that may cause or worsen dementia, such as high blood pressure, high cholesterol, heart disease, diabetes, infections, head injuries, brain tumors, hydrocephalus, anemia, hypoxia, hormone imbalances, and nutritional deficiencies.
- Start low and go slow: psychotropic medication should be used cautiously in elderly and/or neurologically impaired patients. Use lower starting doses, smaller increases in dosage, and longer intervals between increments.
- Behavioral disorders may improve with individualized therapy aimed at identifying and changing specific problem behaviors.
- Agitation should be carefully evaluated to ascertain any reversible causes, such as pain or delirium. Cholinesterase inhibitors can be helpful in some cases. In addition, anticonvulsants may also be helpful. The U.S. Food and Drug Administration issued a warning of a 1.6- to 1.7-fold increase in mortality in elderly patients with dementia who were taking atypical antipsychotics, compared with placebo (Rosack 2005). However, this effect is also

TABLE 8–5.   Pharmacotherapy for dementia

TARGET SYMPTOM(S)	MEDICATION CLASS	STARTING DOSAGE	MAXIMUM DOSAGE
Decreased cognition, delusions, hallucinations	Cholinesterase inhibitors		
	Tacrine	10 mg qid	40 mg qid
	Donepezil	5 mg/day	10 mg/day
	Rivastigmine	1.5 mg bid	6 mg bid
	Galantamine	4 mg bid	12 mg bid
Decreased cognition	Antioxidants		
	Alpha-tocopherol	1,000 IU bid	
	Selegiline	5 mg/day	10 mg/day
Depression, irritability, anxiety	Antidepressants		
Anxiety, irritability	Anxiolytic		
	Buspirone	5 mg tid	20 mg tid
Irritability, agitation	Anticonvulsants		
	Carbamazepine	100 mg/day	[a]
	Valproate	125 mg/day	[b]

TABLE 8–5. Pharmacotherapy for dementia *(continued)*

Target symptom(s)	Medication class	Starting dosage	Maximum dosage
Delusions, hallucinations, disorganized thought, agitation	Antipsychotics		
	Risperidone	0.25 mg/day qhs	3 mg/day qhs
	Olanzapine	2.5 mg/day qhs	10 mg/day qhs
	Quetiapine	25 mg/day qhs	100 mg bid

Note. bid = two times a day; qhs = every bedtime; qid = four times a day; tid = three times a day.
[a]Upper limit of dosage to produce serum drug level of 8–12 ng/mL.
[b]Upper limit of dosage to produce serum drug level of 50–60 ng/mL.
Source. Adapted from Bourgeois et al. 2003.

seen with conventional antipsychotics. Most of the deaths were due to heart-related events (heart failure, sudden death) or infections, primarily pneumonia. As such, nonpsychotic agitation should be treated first with behavior strategies and/or other medications that are not antipsychotics. In psychotic patients, the risk of antipsychotic treatment must be weighed against the potential harm, with family involvement when possible.

References

American Psychiatric Association: Diagnostic and Statistical Manual of Mental Disorders, 4th Edition, Text Revision. Washington, DC, American Psychiatric Association, 2000

American Psychiatric Association: Quick Reference to the American Psychiatric Association Practice Guidelines for the Treatment of Psychiatric Disorders: Compendium 2006. Washington, DC, American Psychiatric Publishing, 2006

Bourgeois JA, Seaman JS, Servis ME: Delirium, dementia, and amnestic disorders, in The American Psychiatric Publishing Textbook of Clinical Psychiatry, 4th Edition. Edited by Hales RE, Yudofsky SC. Washington, DC, American Psychiatric Publishing, 2003, pp 259–308

Cummings JL, Trimble MR: Concise Guide to Neuropsychiatry and Behavioral Neurology, 2nd Edition. Washington, DC, American Psychiatric Publishing, 2002

Lipton AM, Weiner MF: Differential diagnosis, in The Dementias: Diagnosis, Treatment, and Research, 3rd Edition. Edited by Weiner MF, Lipton AM. Washington, DC, American Psychiatric Publishing, 2003, pp 137–180

Rosack J: FDA orders new warning on atypical antipsychotics. Psychiatr News 40:1, 2005

9

Factitious Disorders and Somatoform Disorders

Overview

- *Factitious disorder* is the intentional production of symptoms without external gain.
- *Malingering* is the intentional production of symptoms for external incentives (e.g., to obtain insurance).
- *Somatoform disorders* are not under voluntary control; they were originally designated as "hysteria" and studied extensively by Breuer and Freud.

Assessment is aided by collateral sources such as family members and prior medical records.

Factitious Disorder

Leamon et al. (2007) have described the symptoms and signs of factitious disorder and the common characteristics of patients with this disorder. Table 9–1 presents the DSM-IV-TR (American Psychiatric Association 2000) diagnostic criteria for factitious disorder.

Symptoms of factitious disorder may be subjective (e.g., complaints of abdominal pain), objective but self-inflicted (e.g., self-induced infection of a wound, tampering with lab specimens), or an exaggeration of an existing medical condition (e.g., simulating a grand mal seizure with

---

TABLE 9–1.   DSM-IV-TR diagnostic criteria for factitious disorder

---

A. Intentional production or feigning of physical or psychological signs or symptoms.

B. The motivation for the behavior is to assume the sick role.

C. External incentives for the behavior (such as economic gain, avoiding legal responsibility, or improving physical well-being, as in malingering) are absent.

Code based on type:

> **300.16   With predominantly psychological signs and symptoms:**   if psychological signs and symptoms predominate in the clinical presentation

> **300.19   With predominantly physical signs and symptoms:**   if physical signs and symptoms predominate in the clinical presentation

> **300.19   With combined psychological and physical signs and symptoms:**   if both psychological and physical signs and symptoms are present but neither predominates in the clinical presentation

---

a prior history of a seizure disorder, reporting that mild tension headaches are debilitating).

Common characteristics of patients with factitious disorder:

- Young and female
- Described as passive and immature
- Have health-related jobs or training
- Often report single system complaints

Signs of factitious disorder:

- Discrepancies between objective findings
- Inconsistencies in reported symptoms
- Course of illness may be markedly atypical
- Unusual acquiescence to invasive procedure
- Quarrelsome with staff (especially regarding obtaining previous records)
- Unexplained medical supplies or medications in the patient's possession

Munchausen Syndrome

Munchausen syndrome is a subtype of factitious disorder that is more dramatic and life-threatening. About 10% of factitious disorder cases are considered Munchausen syndrome.

- Patients present with predominantly physical signs and symptoms.
- Patients often present to multiple emergency rooms, with many hospital admissions (Leamon et al. 2003).

Factitious Disorder by Proxy

Factitious disorder by proxy (FDBP), also referred to as *Munchausen by proxy,* often goes undetected. Cases may take months to years to identify; the average time to detection is 14.2 months. Most cases are identified in inpatient medical settings (Rogers 2004).

The following are common signs of FDBP (Leamon et al. 2003):

- One parent (usually the father) is uninvolved.
- The child is taken to multiple care providers.
- The parent is not reassured by normal findings and advocates for invasive or painful tests.
- Signs and symptoms do not occur when the patient is away from the parent.
- Another child in the family has a history of unexplained illness or death.

Table 9–2 presents the DSM-IV-TR research criteria for FDBP.

Differential Diagnosis

- Mood disorders
- Dissociative disorders
- Malingering (in which external motivation is present, such as a patient who presents as psychotic to avoid legal responsibilities)

Treatment

Patients with factitious disorder frequently refuse psychiatric treatment. When treatment is provided, the following guidelines are useful (Leamon et al. 2007):

TABLE 9–2.   DSM-IV-TR research criteria for factitious disorder by proxy

---

A. Intentional production or feigning of physical or psychological signs or symptoms in another person who is under the individual's care.

B. The motivation for the perpetrator's behavior is to assume the sick role by proxy.

C. External incentives for the behavior (such as economic gain) are absent.

D. The behavior is not better accounted for by another mental disorder.

- Use an indirect, nonconfrontational approach.
- Multiple treaters should work together as a team.
- Treat any genuine concomitant illness or comorbid condition (e.g., depression).
- Allow the patient to tacitly give up the factitious symptoms, and do not expect acknowledgment of the deception.
- Psychotherapy may address underlying psychodynamic issues and behavioral strategies may be used, but there is no clinical evidence to support a particular approach.
- Take steps to protect the child and determine legal requirements in cases of abuse.

Malingering

Malingering is the intentional production of false or exaggerated physical or psychological symptoms which is motivated by external gains (e.g., avoiding a legal obligation or gaining economically). Malingering is not considered a mental disorder or psychiatric illness in DSM-IV-TR and is classified under "Other Conditions That May Be a Focus of Clinical Attention" on Axis I.

Signs

Malingering should be suspected if any combination of the following signs is noted (Leamon et al. 2003):

- The individual is referred for evaluation by an attorney.

- The individual's claims do not match objective findings.
- The individual is uncooperative with the evaluation and treatment.
- Antisocial personality disorder is present.

Hallucinations and delusions may be signs of malingering in some cases.

HALLUCINATIONS

- Hallucinations are continuous rather than intermittent.
- Visual hallucinations are in black and white.
- The individual is unable to state strategies to diminish voices.

DELUSIONS

- The individual is eager to discuss delusions.
- The delusions have bizarre content without disorganized thinking.
- The delusions have abrupt onset or termination.
- The individual has elaborate delusions that lack common paranoid, grandiose, or religious themes.

Treatment

In responding to malingering, the clinician may confront the individual in a way that allows the person to save face, for example: "The symptoms you are reporting are not consistent with any known mental illness." However, malingering patients will often be defensive and refuse to accept the diagnosis (Leamon et al. 2007).

Somatoform Disorders

Somatoform disorders include somatization disorder, undifferentiated somatization disorder, conversion disorder, pain disorder, hypochondriasis, and body dysmorphic disorder.

- The physical symptoms suggest physical illness, but there are no known organic findings or physiological mechanisms.
- In contrast to factitious disorder or malingering, somatoform disorder symptoms are not under voluntary control.

Somatization Disorder

Table 9–3 presents the DSM-IV-TR criteria for somatization disorder. This disorder has the following characteristics:

- Multiple unexplained complaints
- Stable over time
- Familial
- Rarely totally remits

DIFFERENTIAL DIAGNOSIS

The following physical disorders may be confused with somatization disorder (Yutzy 2003):

- Multiple sclerosis
- Systemic lupus erythematosus (SLE)
- Acute intermittent porphyria
- Hemochromatosis

The following psychiatric disorders may be confused with somatization disorder (Cloninger 1994):

- Anxiety disorder
- Panic disorder
- Mood disorders (physical symptoms should resolve with treatment of mood disorder)
- Schizophrenia

TREATMENT

Somatization disorder is difficult to treat, and there is a dearth of empirical data to support one treatment over another. It is often treated in the primary care setting.

The following list provides tips for working with a patient with somatization disorder:

- Acknowledge the patient's pain and suffering.
- Communicate to the patient that you are interested in providing care.

TABLE 9–3.   DSM-IV-TR diagnostic criteria for somatization
                  disorder

A. A history of many physical complaints beginning before age 30 years
    that occur over a period of several years and result in treatment being
    sought or significant impairment in social, occupational, or other
    important areas of functioning.

B. Each of the following criteria must have been met, with individual
    symptoms occurring at any time during the course of the disturbance:

    (1) *four pain symptoms:*   a history of pain related to at least four
        different sites or functions (e.g., head, abdomen, back, joints,
        extremities, chest, rectum, during menstruation, during sexual
        intercourse, or during urination)

    (2) *two gastrointestinal symptoms:*   a history of at least two
        gastrointestinal symptoms other than pain (e.g., nausea, bloating,
        vomiting other than during pregnancy, diarrhea, or intolerance of
        several different foods)

    (3) *one sexual symptom:*   a history of at least one sexual or
        reproductive symptom other than pain (e.g., sexual indifference,
        erectile or ejaculatory dysfunction, irregular menses, excessive
        menstrual bleeding, vomiting throughout pregnancy)

    (4) *one pseudoneurological symptom:*   a history of at least one
        symptom or deficit suggesting a neurological condition not
        limited to pain (conversion symptoms such as impaired
        coordination or balance, paralysis or localized weakness, difficulty
        swallowing or lump in throat, aphonia, urinary retention,
        hallucinations, loss of touch or pain sensation, double vision,
        blindness, deafness, seizures; dissociative symptoms such as
        amnesia; or loss of consciousness other than fainting)

C. Either (1) or (2):

    (1) after appropriate investigation, each of the symptoms in criterion
        B cannot be fully explained by a known general medical condition
        or the direct effects of a substance (e.g., a drug of abuse, a
        medication)

TABLE 9–3.   DSM-IV-TR diagnostic criteria for somatization disorder (*continued*)

---

(2) when there is a related general medical condition, the physical complaints or resulting social or occupational impairment are in excess of what would be expected from the history, physical examination, or laboratory findings

D. The symptoms are not intentionally produced or feigned (as in factitious disorder or malingering).

- Inform the patient of the diagnosis without confrontation, and describe it in a positive light.
- Advise the patient that he or she is not "crazy."
- Assure the patient that the possibility of undiscovered physical illness will be assessed on a continuing basis.
- Stress that psychiatric care is supplementary and does not replace medical care.
- Place firm limits on excessive demands, manipulating, or attention seeking.
- Consider regular medical appointments (e.g., 15 minutes every 2 weeks), whether or not a symptom is present. This may give the patient the support needed while not reinforcing the need for symptoms.

Undifferentiated Somatoform Disorder

Table 9–4 presents the DSM-IV-TR diagnostic criteria for undifferentiated somatoform disorder.

DIFFERENTIAL DIAGNOSIS

- Full somatization disorder
- Depression
- Anxiety disorder

TREATMENT

- Supportive psychotherapy may be helpful.
- A substantial number of patients improve with no therapy.
- Anxious and depressive symptoms should be treated.

TABLE 9–4. DSM-IV-TR diagnostic criteria for undifferentiated somatoform disorder

---

A. One or more physical complaints (e.g., fatigue, loss of appetite, gastrointestinal or urinary complaints).

B. Either (1) or (2):

(1) after appropriate investigation, the symptoms cannot be fully explained by a known general medical condition or the direct effects of a substance (e.g., a drug of abuse, a medication)

(2) when there is a related general medical condition, the physical complaints or resulting social or occupational impairment is in excess of what would be expected from the history, physical examination, or laboratory findings

C. The symptoms cause clinically significant distress or impairment in social, occupational, or other important areas of functioning.

D. The duration of the disturbance is at least 6 months.

E. The disturbance is not better accounted for by another mental disorder (e.g., another somatoform disorder, sexual dysfunction, mood disorder, anxiety disorder, sleep disorder, or psychotic disorder).

F. The symptom is not intentionally produced or feigned (as in factitious disorder or malingering).

Conversion Disorder

Patients with conversion disorder present with nonintentional symptoms of deficits affecting voluntary motor or sensory function, such as

- Impaired coordination or balance,
- Paralysis or weakness,
- Blindness or double vision, or
- Seizures with a voluntary motor or sensory component.

Table 9–5 presents the DSM-IV-TR diagnostic criteria for conversion disorder. Symptoms often occur in the context of a conflictual situation. Single episodes usually involve only one system. A narcoanalytic interview (interviewing a patient under the influence of amobarbital) should be used based on case reports only.

TABLE 9–5.   DSM-IV-TR diagnostic criteria for conversion disorder

A.   One or more symptoms or deficits affecting voluntary motor or sensory function that suggest a neurological or other general medical condition.

B.   Psychological factors are judged to be associated with the symptom or deficit because the initiation or exacerbation of the symptom or deficit is preceded by conflicts or other stressors.

C.   The symptom or deficit is not intentionally produced or feigned (as in factitious disorder or malingering).

D.   The symptom or deficit cannot, after appropriate investigation, be fully explained by a general medical condition, or by the direct effects of a substance, or as a culturally sanctioned behavior or experience.

E.   The symptom or deficit causes clinically significant distress or impairment in social, occupational, or other important areas of functioning or warrants medical evaluation.

F.   The symptom or deficit is not limited to pain or sexual dysfunction, does not occur exclusively during the course of somatization disorder, and is not better accounted for by another mental disorder.

Specify type of symptom or deficit:

With motor symptom or deficit

With sensory symptom or deficit

With seizures or convulsions

With mixed presentation

DIFFERENTIAL DIAGNOSIS

- Physical illness (neurological disorder most common)
- Multiple sclerosis
- Myasthenia gravis
- Periodic paralysis
- Myoglobinuric myopathy
- Polymyositis
- Other acquired myopathies
- Guillain-Barré syndrome

TREATMENT

- Work in collaboration with the medical colleague who referred the patient instead of taking a purely psychiatric approach. (Patients with acute conversion disorder most often present to the emergency department or primary care setting.)
- Refer the patient for a complete medical and neurological evaluation. A considerable number of patients initially diagnosed with conversion disorder have undiagnosed medical conditions.
- Work with the patient to develop more adaptive coping skills.
- Treat any comorbid psychiatric disorder.

Pain Disorder

Pain disorder (Table 9–6) is similar to conversion disorder but is more chronic and the symptom is pain (e.g., low back pain, headache, atypical facial pain, chronic pelvic pain). The disorder is seen more often in females. A medical illness may be present but does not adequately account for the degree of pain.

DIFFERENTIAL DIAGNOSIS

- Purely physical pain often fluctuates and is highly sensitive to influence such as emotions and situation.
- Pain that does not wax and wane tends to have a psychogenic component.
- Consider other somatoform disorders (which may be comorbid).

TREATMENT

- Analgesics, nerve blocks, and other surgical treatments are generally not helpful.
- Recognize that the patient's pain experience is real.
- Discuss with the patient how emotional pathways (such as the limbic system and descending spinal pathways) may influence pain perception.
- Agents that affect both serotonin and norepinephrine result in decreased pain perceptions from the periphery. At usual therapeutic dosages, these include amitriptyline, imipramine, and duloxetine. Selective serotonin reuptake inhibitors (SSRIs) are typically not effective in treating physical pain.

TABLE 9–6. DSM-IV-TR diagnostic criteria for pain disorder

A. Pain in one or more anatomical sites is the predominant focus of the clinical presentation and is of sufficient severity to warrant clinical attention.

B. The pain causes clinically significant distress or impairment in social, occupational, or other important areas of functioning.

C. Psychological factors are judged to have an important role in the onset, severity, exacerbation, or maintenance of the pain.

D. The symptom or deficit is not intentionally produced or feigned (as in factitious disorder or malingering).

E. The pain is not better accounted for by a mood, anxiety, or psychotic disorder and does not meet criteria for dyspareunia.

Code as follows:

307.80 Pain disorder associated with psychological factors: psychological factors are judged to have the major role in the onset, severity, exacerbation, or maintenance of the pain. (If a general medical condition is present, it does not have a major role in the onset, severity, exacerbation, or maintenance of the pain.) This type of pain disorder is not diagnosed if criteria are also met for somatization disorder.

Specify if:

Acute: duration of less than 6 months

Chronic: duration of 6 months or longer

307.89 Pain disorder associated with both psychological factors and a general medical condition: both psychological factors and a general medical condition are judged to have important roles in the onset, severity, exacerbation, or maintenance of the pain. The associated general medical condition or anatomical site of the pain (see below) is coded on Axis III.

Specify if:

Acute: duration of less than 6 months

Chronic: duration of 6 months or longer

Note: The following is not considered to be a mental disorder and is included here to facilitate differential diagnosis.

TABLE 9–6. DSM-IV-TR diagnostic criteria for pain
disorder *(continued)*

Pain disorder associated with a general medical condition:
a general medical condition has a major role in the onset, severity,
exacerbation, or maintenance of the pain. (If psychological factors are
present, they are not judged to have a major role in the onset, severity,
exacerbation, or maintenance of the pain.) The diagnostic code for the pain
is selected based on the associated general medical condition if one has
been established, or on the anatomical location of the pain if the underlying
general medical condition is not yet clearly established—for example, low
back (724.2), sciatic (724.3), pelvic (625.9), headache (784.0), facial
(784.0), chest (786.50), joint (719.40), bone (733.90), abdominal (789.0),
breast (611.71), renal (788.0), ear (388.70), eye (379.91), throat (784.1),
tooth (525.9), and urinary (788.0).

- Some data suggest that psychodynamic therapy and more targeted psychotherapies, such as behavioral therapy, including bio-
  feedback, may be helpful.

Hypochondriasis

- Patients with hypochondriasis may have a history of multiple
  complaints without a clear physical basis.
- Fears of aging and death are common.
- Medical history is usually presented at great length.
- Patients often feel as if they are not getting proper care and switch
  doctors frequently.
- Family and social relationships are often strained.

Table 9–7 presents the DSM-IV-TR diagnostic criteria for hypochondriasis.

DIFFERENTIAL DIAGNOSIS

- Neurological diseases (including myasthenia gravis and multiple
  sclerosis)
- Endocrine diseases
- Systemic diseases
- SLE

TABLE 9–7.   DSM-IV-TR diagnostic criteria for hypochondriasis

---

A. Preoccupation with fears of having, or the idea that one has, a serious disease based on the person's misinterpretation of bodily symptoms.

B. The preoccupation persists despite appropriate medical evaluation and reassurance.

C. The belief in criterion A is not of delusional intensity (as in delusional disorder, somatic type) and is not restricted to a circumscribed concern about appearance (as in body dysmorphic disorder).

D. The preoccupation causes clinically significant distress or impairment in social, occupational, or other important areas of functioning.

E. The duration of the disturbance is at least 6 months.

F. The preoccupation is not better accounted for by generalized anxiety disorder, obsessive-compulsive disorder, panic disorder, a major depressive episode, separation anxiety, or another somatoform disorder.

Specify if:

With poor insight: if, for most of the time during the current episode, the person does not recognize that the concern about having a serious illness is excessive or unreasonable

---

- Malignancies
- Generalized anxiety disorder
- Anxiety disorder
- Delusional disorder
  - Schizophrenia: Patients with schizophrenia will show other signs of schizophrenia, such as peculiar thoughts and behavior and hallucinations.
  - Hypochondriasis: Patients with hypochondriasis are generally able to acknowledge that concerns are unfounded.

TREATMENT

- Emphasize that psychiatric involvement is a supplement to, not a replacement for, continued medical care.
- Hospitalizations, medical tests, and addictive medications are to be avoided.

- The focus of supportive therapy should shift from symptoms to social or interpersonal problems. No evidence supports one method of therapy as superior to another.
- Treat any comorbid psychiatric disorder.
- Consider regular medical appointments (e.g., 15 minutes every 2 weeks), whether or not a symptom is present. This may give the patient the support needed while not reinforcing the need for symptoms.

Body Dysmorphic Disorder

The essential feature of body dysmorphic disorder (Table 9–8) is a preoccupation with an imagined defect in physical appearance or an exaggeration of minor physical anomaly such as flaws of face or head (e.g., defects in hair [too much or too little], skin, shape of face, nose, ears); flaws of body parts (e.g., genitals, breasts, buttocks, shoulders); and/or overall body size. This disorder is commonly seen among people seeking cosmetic surgery.

DIFFERENTIAL DIAGNOSIS

- Anorexia nervosa
- Gender identity disorder
- Major depression
- Obsessive-compulsive disorder
- Delusional disorder

TABLE 9–8. DSM-IV-TR diagnostic criteria for body dysmorphic disorder

---

A. Preoccupation with an imagined defect in appearance. If a slight physical anomaly is present, the person's concern is markedly excessive.

B. The preoccupation causes clinically significant distress or impairment in social, occupational, or other important areas of functioning.

C. The preoccupation is not better accounted for by another mental disorder (e.g., dissatisfaction with body shape and size in anorexia nervosa).

TREATMENT

- Antidepressants, especially SSRIs at a relatively high dose for at least 12 weeks' duration, may be helpful.

- Cognitive-behavioral therapy, consisting of elements such as exposure, response prevention, behavioral experiments, and cognitive restructuring, may be beneficial. Other psychotherapies are not well studied but have some support in the form of case reports.

- There is no evidence to support that surgery to correct the physical flaw is helpful.

References

American Psychiatric Association: Diagnostic and Statistical Manual of Mental Disorders, 4th Edition, Text Revision. Washington, DC, American Psychiatric Association, 2000

Cloninger CR: Somatoform and dissociative disorders, in The Medical Basis of Psychiatry, 2nd Edition. Edited by Winokur G, Clayton PJ. Philadelphia, PA, WB Saunders, 1994, pp 169–192

Leamon MH, Feldman MD, Scott CL: Factitious disorders and malingering, in The American Psychiatric Publishing Textbook of Clinical Psychiatry, 4th Edition. Edited by Hales RE, Yudofsky SC. Washington, DC, American Psychiatric Publishing, 2003, pp 691–707

Leamon MH, Feldman MD, Scott CL: Factitious disorders and malingering, in Board Prep and Review Course for Psychiatry. Edited by Bourgeois JA, Hales RE, Yudofsky SC. Washington, DC, American Psychiatric Publishing, 2007, pp 245–249

Rogers R: Diagnostic, explanatory, and detection models of Munchausen by proxy: extrapolations from malingering and deception. Child Abuse Negl 28:225–239, 2004

Yutzy SH: Somatoform disorders, in The American Psychiatric Publishing Textbook of Clinical Psychiatry, 4th Edition. Edited by Hales RE, Yudofsky SC. Washington, DC, American Psychiatric Publishing, 2003, pp 659–690

10

Eating Disorders

Anorexia nervosa and bulimia nervosa are most common in females, with more than 90% of anorexia nervosa cases occurring in females. The lifetime prevalence in females is approximately 0.5% for anorexia nervosa and 1%–3% for bulimia nervosa (American Psychiatric Association 2000).

Assessments

The American Psychiatric Association (2006) Practice Guideline lists assessments for patients with eating disorders.

History

- Weight and weight history
- Restrictive and binge eating
- Exercise patterns (may tend to stand vs. sit; may generate opportunities to be physically active; may be drawn to sports, athletics, and dance)
- Purging behaviors (e.g., vomiting, use of laxatives or diuretics)
- Attitudes regarding weight, shape, and eating
- Obsessive behavior (e.g., frequent weighing, checking in mirror)
- Family history of eating disorders and obesity

General Medical Condition (Baseline and Ongoing)

- Blood pressure (including orthostatic)
- Pulse
- Oral temperature
- Other cardiovascular parameters
- Height and weight (weight taken after voiding with patient in a hospital gown)
- Body mass index (BMI)
- Dental examination referral
- Bone density exam (for patients who are amenorrheic for 6 months or more)
- Electrolytes

In younger patients, growth pattern and sexual development should also be assessed. Table 10–1 lists suggested laboratory assessments for patients with eating disorders.

Anorexia Nervosa

Table 10–2 presents the DSM-IV-TR (American Psychiatric Association 2000) diagnostic criteria for anorexia nervosa. Morris and Twaddle (2007) have described the features of this disorder:

- Onset is typically with onset of puberty and adolescence.
- There is a premorbid preoccupation with physical appearance and weight.
- Unusual interactions with food are common, such as cutting food into very small pieces, hoarding food but not eating it, and cooking meals for others but not participating in eating the meal.
- Excessive exercise is common.
- Weight loss is often concealed.
- Common medical complications include amenorrhea, potassium depletion, cardiac arrest, and osteoporosis.

TABLE 10–1. Suggested laboratory assessments for patients with eating disorders

ASSESSMENT	PATIENT INDICATION
Basic analyses	For all patients with eating disorders
Blood chemistry studies	
Serum electrolytes	
Blood urea nitrogen (BUN)	
Serum creatinine (interpretations must incorporate assessments of weight)	
Thyroid-stimulating hormone (TSH); if indicated free T_4, T_3	
Complete blood cell count (CBC), including differential and erythrocyte sedimentation rate	
Aspartate aminotransferase (AST), alanine aminotransferase (ALT), alkaline phosphatase (ALP)	
Urinalysis	

TABLE 10–1. Suggested laboratory assessments for patients with eating disorders *(continued)*

ASSESSMENT	PATIENT INDICATION
Additional analyses	
Complement component C3[a]	For malnourished and severely symptomatic patients. Serum magnesium should be obtained prior to beginning certain medications if QTc is prolonged. *Note:* During hospital refeeding, serum potassium, magnesium, and phosphorus should be followed daily for 5 days and thereafter at least three times a week for 3 weeks.
Blood chemistry studies	
Serum calcium	
Serum magnesium	
Serum ferritin	
Electrocardiogram	
24-Hour urine for creatinine clearance[b]	
Osteopenia and osteoporosis assessments	For patients with amenorrhea of more than 6 months' duration
Dual energy X-ray absorptiometry (DEXA)	
Serum estradiol in females	
Serum testosterone in males	

TABLE 10–1. Suggested laboratory assessments for patients with eating disorders *(continued)*

ASSESSMENT	PATIENT INDICATION
Nonroutine assessments	
Drug screen	For patients with suspected substance abuse, particularly patients with anorexia nervosa, binge/purge subtype, or bulimia nervosa
Serum amylase (fractionated for salivary gland isoenzyme if available, to rule out pancreatic involvement)	
Serum luteinizing hormone (LH), follicle-stimulating hormone (FSH); β-human chorionic gonadotropin (HCG) and prolactin	For patients with persistent amenorrhea at normal weight
Brain magnetic resonance imaging (MRI) and computed tomography (CT)	For patients with significant cognitive deficits, other neurological soft signs, unremitting course, or other atypical features
Stool for guaiac	For patients with suspected gastrointestinal bleeding
Stool or urine for bisacodyl, emodin, aloe-emodin, rhein	For patients with suspected laxative abuse

Note. T₃=triiodothyronine; T₄=thyroxine.

ᵃSome experts recommend the routine use of complement component C3 as a sensitive marker that may indicate nutritional deficiencies even when other laboratory test results are apparently normal (Nova et al. 2004; Wyatt et al. 1982).

ᵇBoag et al. 1985. Creatinine clearance should be calculated using equations that involve body surface based on assessments of height and weight.

Source. Adapted from Yager 2007.

TABLE 10–2.   DSM-IV-TR criteria for anorexia nervosa

A. Refusal to maintain body weight at or above a minimally normal weight for age and height (e.g., weight loss leading to maintenance of body weight less than 85% of that expected; or failure to make expected weight gain during period of growth, leading to body weight less than 85% of that expected).

B. Intense fear of gaining weight or becoming fat, even though underweight.

C. Disturbance in the way in which one's body weight or shape is experienced, undue influence of body weight or shape on self-evaluation, or denial of the seriousness of the current low body weight.

D. In postmenarcheal females, amenorrhea, i.e., the absence of at least three consecutive menstrual cycles. (A woman is considered to have amenorrhea if her periods occur only following hormone, e.g., estrogen, administration.)

Specify type:

Restricting type: during the current episode of anorexia nervosa, the person has not regularly engaged in binge-eating or purging behavior (i.e., self-induced vomiting or the misuse of laxatives, diuretics, or enemas)

Binge-eating/purging type: during the current episode of anorexia nervosa, the person has regularly engaged in binge-eating or purging behavior (i.e., self-induced vomiting or the misuse of laxatives, diuretics, or enemas)

Course

- 50% achieve full recovery.
- 30% improve.
- 20% remain chronically ill.
- 50% will also develop bulimic symptoms.
- 1 out of 3 patients who recover will relapse.
- Mortality is due to suicide or cardiac failure.

Differential Diagnosis

- Healthy dieting to lose weight is not accompanied by amenorrhea or other signs of adverse physiological effects.

- Anorexia nervosa typically manifests in adolescence; midlife onset is rare. Especially in older patients, it is important to rule out other medical conditions (Herzog and Eddy 2007):
  - Diabetes mellitus
  - Colitis
  - Thyroid disease
  - Inflammatory bowel disease
  - Acid peptic disease
  - Addison disease
  - Intestinal motility disorder
  - Brain tumor

Treatment

Patients with anorexia should be referred for individual and family therapy with a component of cognitive-behavioral therapy (CBT). Family involvement is important. Family interactions and attitudes toward eating, exercise, and appearance have an impact on eating disorders. Group therapy can also be helpful.

Resistance to treatment is common. Involuntary hospitalization or establishment of legal guardianship may be needed if the patient's medical condition is life-threatening.

MEDICATIONS

Selective serotonin reuptake inhibitors (SSRIs) are commonly used in combination with psychotherapy and may be helpful in treating depressive, anxiety, or obsessive-compulsive symptoms. However, recent data suggest that the use of an SSRI following weight restoration does not reduce the risk of relapse (Walsh et al. 2006). Bupropion should not be used in patients with eating disorders, because of the increased risk of seizures. Calcium and vitamin D supplements are often recommended as well as multivitamins containing zinc, which may accelerate an increase in weight (American Psychiatric Association 2006; Bulik et al. 2007).

TREATMENT SETTING

While weight and BMI are important indicators of eating disorders, they should not be the sole indicators of physical risk. According to the American Psychiatric Association (2006) Practice Guideline, the most important factors regarding the patient's overall physical condition to consider when choosing a treatment setting are

- Weight in relation to estimated individually healthy weight,
- Rate of weight loss,
- Cardiac function, and
- Metabolic status.

There are a wide range of treatment settings for eating disorders, and specialized programs are not available in all areas. Evidence suggests that inpatient settings with staff experienced in eating disorders have improved outcomes compared with general inpatient units with inexperienced staff.

The American Psychiatric Association Practice Guideline (2006) sets the following target goals for weight gain: 2–3 pounds per week inpatient setting and 0.5–1 pound per week for outpatient setting.

Bulimia Nervosa

- Onset is typically in adolescence after attempts at dieting.
- About one-quarter of patients with bulimia nervosa have previously been diagnosed with anorexia nervosa (American Psychiatric Association 2006).
- It is frequently comorbid with other disorders, especially mood and anxiety disorders, personality disorders, and substance abuse.
- A key feature is binge eating.
- Self-induced vomiting, laxatives, and diuretics may be used after a binge. Look for abrasions on the back of the hand and enamel erosion on the teeth from self-induced vomiting.
- Common medical complications include dental complications, potassium depletion, increased amylase, salivary gland enlargement, and arrhythmias.
- Mortality is not increased in bulimia nervosa, in contrast to anorexia nervosa.

Table 10–3 presents the DSM-IV-TR diagnostic criteria for bulimia nervosa.

TABLE 10–3.   DSM-IV-TR criteria for bulimia nervosa

A.   Recurrent episodes of binge eating. An episode of binge eating is characterized by both of the following:

   (1) eating, in a discrete period of time (e.g., within any 2-hour period), an amount of food that is definitely larger than most people would eat during a similar period of time and under similar circumstances

   (2) a sense of lack of control over eating during the episode (e.g., a feeling that one cannot stop eating or control what or how much one is eating)

B.   Recurrent inappropriate compensatory behavior in order to prevent weight gain, such as self-induced vomiting; misuse of laxatives, diuretics, enemas, or other medications; fasting; or excessive exercise.

C.   The binge eating and inappropriate compensatory behaviors both occur, on average, at least twice a week for 3 months.

D.   Self-evaluation is unduly influenced by body shape and weight.

E.   The disturbance does not occur exclusively during episodes of anorexia nervosa.

Specify type:

   Purging type: during the current episode of bulimia nervosa, the person has regularly engaged in self-induced vomiting or the misuse of laxatives, diuretics, or enemas

   Nonpurging type: during the current episode of bulimia nervosa, the person has used other inappropriate compensatory behaviors, such as fasting or excessive exercise, but has not regularly engaged in self-induced vomiting or the misuse of laxatives, diuretics, or enemas

---

Differential Diagnosis

- Anorexic patients may also binge eat and purge.
- Binge-eating disorder includes eating binges but not compensatory behaviors, such as purging or excessive exercise.
- Consider neurological disorders:
  - Brain tumors (e.g., pituitary, hypothalamic)
  - Kleine-Levin syndrome (excessive amounts of sleep, excessive food intake, and uninhibited sexual drive)

- Klüver-Bucy syndrome (urge to put all kinds of objects into the mouth, memory loss, extreme sexual behavior, placidity, and visual distractibility)

- Consider gastrointestinal disorders:
  - Malabsorption
  - Ulcers
  - Enteritis

Treatment

Evidence supports that CBT is the most effective single intervention. Therapy may be individual or group. Most patients with bulimia need a combination of CBT and antidepressant medication. Fluoxetine is the best studied, but other SSRIs are likely effective.

References

American Psychiatric Association: Diagnostic and Statistical Manual of Mental Disorders, 4th Edition, Text Revision. Washington, DC, American Psychiatric Association, 2000

American Psychiatric Association: Treatment of patients with eating disorders, third edition. American Psychiatric Association. Am J Psychiatry 163 (suppl 7):4–54, 2006

Boag F, Weerakoon J, Ginsburg J, et al: Diminished creatinine clearance in anorexia nervosa: reversal with weight gain. J Clin Pathol 38:60–63, 1985

Bulik CM, Berkman ND, Brownley KA, et al: Anorexia nervosa treatment: a systematic review of randomized controlled trials. Int J Eat Disord 40:310-320, 2007

Herzog DB, Eddy KT: Diagnosis, epidemiology, and clinical course of eating disorders, in Clinical Manual of Eating Disorders. Edited by Yager J, Powers PS. Washington, DC, American Psychiatric Publishing, 2007, pp 1–29

Morris J, Twaddle S: Anorexia nervosa. BMJ 334:894–898, 2007

Nova E, Lopez-Vidriero I, Varela O, et al: Indicators of nutritional status in restricting-type anorexia nervosa patients: a 1-year follow-up study. Clin Nutr 23:1353–1359, 2004

Walsh BT, Kaplan AS, Attia E, et al: Fluoxetine after weight restoration in anorexia nervosa: a randomized controlled trial. JAMA 295:2605–2612, 2006

Wyatt RJ, Farrell M, Berry PL, et al: Reduced alternative complement pathway control protein levels in anorexia nervosa: response to parenteral alimentation. Am J Clin Nutr 35:973–980, 1982

Yager J: Assessment and determination of initial treatment approaches for patients with eating disorders, in Clinical Manual of Eating Disorders. Edited by Yager J, Powers PS. Washington, DC, American Psychiatric Publishing, 2007, pp 31–77

11

Consultation-Liaison Psychiatry

Consultation-liaison psychiatry refers to a psychiatrist rendering care in a medical setting, such as an inpatient medical or surgical unit, a medical emergency room, or an outpatient medical/surgical clinic. The goals are to offer an opinion regarding diagnosis and treatment of psychiatric or behavior problems, to ensure the safety and stability of the patient within a medical environment, and to educate the staff regarding problems that may arise from managing a psychotic, agitated, or manipulative patient within a medical or surgical environment.

Consultation Documentation

The development of the medical-psychiatric history should include a physical/neurological and mental status examination. The consultation note should synthesize the data, provide a diagnosis, and recommend appropriate testing and treatment. The following areas may need special inquiry (Bronheim et al. 1998):

- *Reason for referral.* The consultee-stated versus consultant-assessed reason for referral should be clarified.
- *Medical/surgical illness.* Many patients have complex medical conditions, so the medical chart should be reviewed for pertinent medical factors that could contribute to their current state.
- *Pain management.* It is important to conduct a detailed assessment of all analgesics and adjunctive medications. It is essential to

have an awareness of how pain contributes to specific illnesses, as well as how psychiatric disorders and symptoms contribute to pain complaints and vice versa (e.g., anxiety in acute pain, depression in chronic pain).

- *Medications or substance abuse.*   Psychiatric symptoms are frequently caused by medications prescribed for medical disorders. Analgesics, sedatives, anticonvulsants, anesthetics, psychotropics, and anticholinergics are commonly associated with psychiatric symptoms (see Table 11–1).

- *Disturbances in cognition.*   Determine if the change in mental status is chronic and due to the underlying disorder (e.g., Alzheimer's disease) or acute (e.g., delirium) and occurring secondary to the effects of illness, medication, or a combination of factors, typically with a waxing and waning course.

- *Psychiatric symptomatology and behavior.*   Consider whether the behavior is a normal response to the stress of illness and/or hospitalization. Explore prior response to illness or psychiatric treatment.

Competency and Capacity for Health Care Decision Making

Competency is a legal term; the designation of competency is made by the courts, not by a psychiatrist. A patient deemed incompetent by the courts will have a legal guardian.

A legally incompetent patient may not choose to give informed consent. In an emergency where the guardian is not readily available, document this fact as well as the risk to the patient of not rendering immediate treatment, and contact the hospital administrator and the patient's family.

Although the consulting physician asks you to evaluate competency, what you are actually doing is assessing the patient's capacity to make an informed decision. The assessment of capacity includes

- Communication of choice,
- Understanding of relevant information provided,
- Appreciation of available options and consequences, and
- Rational decision making (note that just because you do not agree with the patient does not mean that the choice is not rational [Simon and Shuman 2007]).

TABLE 11–1. Medical disorders that commonly cause or exacerbate psychiatric symptoms

SUBSTANCE ABUSE AND MEDICATION TOXICITY	CNS DISORDERS	INFECTIONS	METABOLIC/ ENDOCRINE DISORDERS	CARDIOPULMONARY DISORDERS	MISCELLANEOUS
Alcohol/drug abuse	CNS infection	Acute rheumatic fever	Adrenal disease	Arrhythmias	Anemia
Amphetamines	Hypertensive encephalopathy	Hepatitis	Electrolyte imbalances	Asthma	Lupus
Anabolic steroids	Intracranial aneurysm	Pneumonia	Hepatic encephalopathy	Congestive heart failure	NMS
Benzodiazepines	Migraine headache	Sepsis	Renal disease	COPD	Serotonin syndrome
Cocaine	Normal-pressure hydrocephalus	Syphilis	Thyroid disease	Myocardial infarction	Temporal arteritis
Ecstasy	Seizures	Urinary tract infection	Vitamin deficiencies	Pulmonary embolism	Vasculitis
Heroin	Subdural hematoma				
LSD	Tumor				
PCP					
THC					
Prescription drugs					

Note. CNS=central nervous system; COPD=chronic obstructive pulmonary disease; LSD=lysergic acid diethylamide; NMS=neuroleptic malignant syndrome; PCP=phencyclidine; THC=Δ-tetrahydrocannabinol.
Source. Adapted from Williams and Shepherd 2000.

Delirium

Delirium is an acute, potentially reversible change in cognition, which may include memory impairment, disorientation, or language disturbance or development of a perceptual disturbance. Table 11–2 summarizes the prevalence of delirium. The following are key features of delirium (see Table 11–3 for more detail):

- The disturbance develops over a short period of time and tends to fluctuate during the course of the day—that is, waxing and waning mental status (e.g., the person may be coherent and cooperative earlier in the day, but at night might insist on pulling out intravenous lines and going home to parents who died years ago).
- The ability to focus, sustain, or shift attention is impaired.
- Evidence from the history, physical examination, or laboratory tests indicates that the delirium is a direct physiological consequence of a general medical condition, substance intoxication or withdrawal, use of a medication (Table 11–4), toxin exposure, or a combination of these factors.
- The typical course of delirium is 10–12 days, but it can range from 1 week to 2 months.

TABLE 11–2.   Prevalence of delirium

POPULATION	PREVALENCE (%)
In general population ages 18 years and older	0.4
In general population ages 55 years and older	1.1
In hospitalized medically ill	10–30
In hospitalized elderly	10–40
In nursing home residents and those ages 75 years and older	Up to 60
In hospitalized patients with cancer	Up to 25
In hospitalized patients with AIDS	30–40
In terminal illness near death	Up to 80

Note.   Rates in these populations vary depending on medical condition.
Source.   Data from American Psychiatric Association 2000.

TABLE 11–3. Clinical features of delirium

Attention deficits	Questions must be repeated because the individual's attention wanders.
	Patient may be easily distracted by irrelevant stimuli.
	It may be difficult (or impossible) to engage the person in conversation.
Memory impairment	Patient cannot register new information.
	Ask patient to remember several unrelated objects or a brief sentence and have them repeat after a few minutes of distraction.
Disorientation	This may be the first symptom to appear.
	Patient is usually disoriented to time and/or place.
	Disorientation to self is less common.
Speech or language impairments	Speech may be rambling, irrelevant, pressured, and/or incoherent.
	Dysarthria: impaired ability to articulate
	Dysnomia: impaired ability to name objects
	Dysgraphia: impaired ability to write
	Aphasia: impaired language comprehension and production
Perceptual disturbances	Misinterpretations, illusions, or hallucinations
	Visual misinterpretations are most common.
	There may be delusional conviction of the reality of the hallucination, along with emotional and behavioral responses.
Fluctuating course	Prodrome (restlessness, anxiety, sleep disturbance, irritability)
	Acute onset
	Changing symptoms

Source.   Adapted from Hilty et al. 2007.

TABLE 11–4.   Selected psychiatric side effects of medications

CLASS/DRUG	EFFECTS
Anticonvulsants	
Vigabatrin	Agitation, lethargy, irritability, agitation, major depression, psychosis ("schizophrenia-like," in 2%–4% of treated patients), cognitive impairment
Topiramate	Psychosis (6% of treated patients), depression, emotional lability, cognitive difficulties
Tiagabine	Psychosis (0.8% of treated patients), depressive symptoms, sedation
Levetiracetam	Irritability, sedation, psychosis
Anti-infectives	
Cycloserine	Dose-dependent side effects: depression, irritability (common), psychosis
Isoniazid	Cognitive impairment, mood disorder, psychosis
Acyclovir	Lethargy, psychosis
Foscarnet sodium	Fatigue, mood changes, psychosis, dementia
Ganciclovir	Sleep disturbances, anxiety, mood disorders, psychosis
Amphotericin B	Delirium
Ketoconazole	Decreased libido, mood disorders, psychosis
Griseofulvin	Depression, psychosis, sleep disturbances
Chloroquine, mefloquine	Anxiety, depression, suicidality, panic attacks, hallucinations, psychosis

TABLE 11–4. Selected psychiatric side effects of medications *(continued)*

CLASS/DRUG	EFFECTS
Anti-infectives *(continued)*	
Quinine	Cinchonism (including vertigo, altered color perception, anxiety, confusion, delirium)
Corticosteroids	Lethargy, sleep disturbances, anxiety, agitation, euphoria, depression, personality changes, psychological dependence, psychosis, delirium
Cyclosporine A	Anxiety, depression, psychosis, cognitive impairment, delirium
Interferon (α and β)	Sleep disturbance, depression, suicidal ideation, cognitive impairment, delirium
Methotrexate	Personality changes, irritability, delirium
Antineoplastic agents	
Interferon, L-asparaginase, interleukin, isophosphamide, methotrexate, vinblastine, vincristine	Delirium, lethargy, hallucinations, depression, psychosis
Antiparkinsonian medications	
L-Dopa (carbidopa or benserazide combinations)	Visual hallucinations, depression, hypomania, sleep disturbance, abnormal dreams, cognitive impairment, psychosis, agitation, delirium

TABLE 11–4. Selected psychiatric side effects of medications *(continued)*

CLASS/DRUG	EFFECTS
Antiparkinsonian medications *(continued)*	
Apomorphine, bromocriptine, cabergoline, lisuride, pergolide, ropinirole, pramipexole	Sedation, psychomotor agitation, anxiety, akathisia, sleep disturbance, hallucinations, psychosis, cognitive impairment, delirium
Selegiline	Sleep disturbances, agitation, psychosis
Entacapone	Sleep disturbances, hallucinations, delirium
Cardiovascular medications	
Digoxin	Visual hallucinations (classically, yellow rings around objects), delirium, depression
Beta-blockers	Fatigue, sexual dysfunction more common than depression per se, possibly less effect with atenolol
Methyldopa	Depression, confusion, insomnia
Clonidine	Depression

Source. Adapted from Turjanski and Lloyd 2005.

Assessment

The following assessments should be performed in a patient presenting with symptoms of delirium (Hilty et al. 2007):

PHYSICAL STATUS

- History
- General physical and neurological examinations
- Review of vital signs and anesthesia record if postoperative
- Review of general medical and psychiatric records
- Careful review of medications, medication interactions, and correlation with behavioral changes

MENTAL STATUS

- Interview with patient
- Interview with family members and/or nursing staff
- Cognitive tests (e.g., clock face, digit span, Trail Making Test)

BASIC LABORATORY TESTS

These tests should be considered for all patients with delirium.

- Blood chemistries: electrolytes, glucose, calcium, albumin, blood urea nitrogen (BUN), creatinine, AST, ALT, bilirubin, alkaline phosphatase, magnesium, phosphorus
- Complete blood cell count (CBC)
- Electrocardiogram
- Chest X ray
- Arterial blood gases or oxygen saturation
- Urinalysis

ADDITIONAL LABORATORY TESTS

These additional tests should be ordered as indicated by clinical condition.

- Urine culture and sensitivity (C&S)
- Urine drug screen

- Blood tests (e.g., Venereal Disease Research Laboratory [VDRL], heavy metal screen, vitamin B_{12} and folate levels, antinuclear antibody [ANA], urinary porphyrins, ammonia level, HIV, erythrocyte sedimentation rate [ESR])
- Blood cultures
- Serum levels of medications (e.g., digoxin, theophylline, phenobarbital, cyclosporine)
- Lumbar puncture
- Brain computed tomography or magnetic resonance imaging
- Electroencephalogram (EEG)

Differential Diagnosis

It is important to differentiate delirium from dementia, which has a more subtle onset and chronic memory and executive function distur-

TABLE 11–5.   Differential diagnosis for delirium: WITCHED-TM

Withdrawal	Alcohol, barbiturates, sedative-hypnotics, Wernicke's encephalopathy, Korsakoff's syndrome
Infectious	Encephalitis, meningitis, abscesses, syphilis
Trauma	Head trauma, heat stroke, surgery, severe burns
CNS pathology	Normal-pressure hydrocephalus, seizures, tumors, hypertensive encephalopathy, bleeds, shock, inflammation/vasculitis
Hypoxia	Anemia, carbon monoxide poisoning, hypotension, pulmonary or cardiac failure
Endocrinopathies	Hyper- or hypoadrenocorticism, hyper- or hypoglycemia, others
Deficiencies	Vitamin B_{12}, niacin, thiamine, hypovitaminosis
Toxins or drugs	Medications, pesticides, solvents, other toxic agents (lead, manganese, mercury), over-the-counter medications, anticholinergic medications
Metabolic	Acidosis, alkalosis, electrolyte disturbance, hepatic failure, renal failure

Note.   CNS=central nervous system.
Source.   Adapted from Hilty et al. 2007.

bances. Also, patients with dementia have impoverished speech and thinking, as opposed to the confused or disorganized speech seen in delirium. Patients with dementia are more likely to have a consistent mental status throughout the day. Table 11–5 explains the differential diagnosis mnemonic WITCHED-TM.

Treatment

Table 11–6 presents examples of reversible causes of delirium and their treatments.

The following are general guidelines for treating a patient with delirium or agitation:

1. Prevent injury; clear the area.
2. Restrain the patient if necessary to prevent harm to self or others (see guidelines for documentation in Chapter 1, "Assessment and Documentation").
3. Look for the basic etiology (e.g., delirium, pain, psychosis).
4. Identify situational stressors that can be mitigated.
5. Treat the patient pharmacologically if appropriate.
   a. Use an atypical antipsychotic, such as olanzapine 10 mg po or im, or ziprasidone 10–20 mg im (up to 40 mg/day), or the typical antipsychotic haloperidol 5 mg po or im. Watch for extrapyramidal side effects. Use caution with patients diagnosed with Alzheimer's disease.
   b. Alternate with lorazepam 1–2 mg po or im every 2–4 hours, if not intoxicated with alcohol or barbiturates. Use lower doses in the medically ill and elderly. Watch for paradoxical agitation. Watch for respiratory depression in patients who are already in poor respiratory status (otherwise, respiratory depression is very rare).
6. Provide for the patient's ongoing treatment and safety.

Fibromyalgia

The American College of Rheumatology criteria for fibromyalgia are as follows (Wolfe 1990):

1. History of widespread pain of at least 3 months' duration. *Widespread* means pain in the right and left side of the body, pain above and below the waist, and axial skeletal pain (cervical spine or ante-

TABLE 11–6. **Examples of reversible causes of delirium and their treatments**

Condition	Treatment
Hypoglycemia or delirium of unknown etiology in which hypoglycemia is suspected	Tests of blood (usually finger stick to establish diagnosis Thiamine hydrochloride, 100 mg iv (before glucose) 50% glucose solution, 50 mL iv
Hypoxia or anoxia (e.g., due to pneumonia, obstructive or restrictive pulmonary disease, cardiac disease, hypertension, severe anemia, or carbon monoxide poisoning)	Immediate oxygen
Hyperthermia (e.g., temperature above 40.5°C or 105°F)	Rapid cooling
Severe hypertension (e.g., blood pressure of 260/150 mm Hg, with papilledema)	Prompt antihypertensive treatment
Alcohol or sedative withdrawal	Appropriate pharmacological intervention
	Thiamine, intravenous glucose, magnesium, phosphate, and other B vitamins, including folate
Wernicke's encephalopathy	Thiamine hydrochloride, 100 mg iv, followed by thiamine daily, either intravenously or orally
Anticholinergic delirium	Withdrawal of offending agent
	In severe cases, physostigmine should be considered unless contraindicated.

Note.   iv=intravenously.
Source.   Adapted from American Psychiatric Association 2006.

rior chest or thoracic spine or low back). In this definition, shoulder and buttock pain is considered as pain for each involved side. *Low back pain* is considered lower-segment pain.

2. Pain, on digital palpation, must be present in at least 11–18 specified tender point sites. Digital palpation should be performed with an approximate force of 4 kg. For a tender point to be considered "positive," the patient must state that the palpation was painful.

While fibromyalgia is a condition produced by central pain sensitization, patients with fibromyalgia are often difficult to diagnose, and therefore psychiatric consultations are sought. Table 11–7 presents the medical differential diagnosis for patients with chronic fatigue syndrome and fibromyalgia syndrome. Information about treatment is rapidly evolving. Medications with FDA approval for treatment of fibromyalgia specifically include pregabalin and duloxetine.

Treatment of Psychiatric Disorders in the Medical Setting

Patients With Hepatic Disease

- Whenever possible, avoid psychotropic medications that require extensive first-pass metabolism, such as bupropion, quetiapine, sertraline, or venlafaxine. Duloxetine is not recommended in patients with known liver disease.

- Medications that only require glucuronidation (temazepam, oxazepam, and lorazepam) are preferred to drugs that require oxidation.

- As a general rule of thumb, decrease the dose of psychotropics metabolized by the liver by 50% in moderate liver disease and by 75% in severe liver disease. Although lithium is excreted unchanged by the kidneys, it may be difficult to manage due to changes in fluid shifts and renal function in patients with liver disease, especially cirrhosis (Crone et al. 2006).

Patients With Renal Disease

- While some sources recommend that patients with renal disease receive two-thirds the ordinary or maximum dose of most psychotropic medications, Cohen et al. (2004) found that most patients with renal disease tolerate and require ordinary doses.

TABLE 11–7. Medical differential diagnosis for patients with chronic fatigue syndrome (CFS) and fibromyalgia syndrome (FMS)

Diagnosis	Syndrome	Differentiating clinical features	Initial workup
Thyroid disorders	CFS, FMS	Hypothyroidism: cold intolerance, slowed relaxation phase of reflexes, weight gain, elevated cholesterol	Thyrotropin
		Hyperthyroidism: heat intolerance, tremor, weight loss	
Medications (statins)	CFS, FMS	Symptom resolution with withdrawal of medication	Creatine kinase, aldolase
Sleep apnea	CFS, FMS	Daytime somnolence, motor vehicle accidents, witnessed nighttime apnea and snoring, hypertension	Sleep study
Spinal stenosis	FMS	History of osteoarthritis, degenerative disc disease, back pain with radiculopathy, sensory and /or motor deficits, pseudoclaudication	Nerve conduction study, electromyogram, MRI of spine if neurological deficits
Anemia	CFS	Pallor	Complete blood cell count

Note. MRI=magnetic resonance imaging.
Source. Adapted from Sharpe and O'Mally 2007.

- The newer antipsychotics, such as olanzapine and ziprasidone, are probably best avoided in patients with renal disease. For the management of agitation/delirium, use a traditional antipsychotic, such as haloperidol. Less than 1% of haloperidol is excreted in the urine, and it appears to be safe in patients with renal disease (Cohen et al. 2004).
- Benzodiazepines are metabolized in the liver, so dose reduction is not usually necessary in patients with renal disease (Cohen et al. 2004).
- Selective serotonin reuptake inhibitors appear to be tolerated by patients with renal disease. Fluoxetine is the best studied, and renal function does not significantly alter serum levels of fluoxetine or norfluoxetine. Sertraline is also commonly used and is metabolized by the liver. Citalopram kinetics are similar and appear to be minimally changed in patients with renal disease. However, plasma concentrations of paroxetine are increased in patients with renal impairment, and the recommended initial dose should be halved (Cohen et al. 2004).
- Divalproex and carbamazepine may be useful in patients with renal disease, but free serum levels of valproic acid may become elevated. If lithium is necessary, dosing should occur after dialysis (Cohen et al. 2004).

Cardiac Side Effects of Psychotropic Drugs

Psychotropic drugs can have cardiac side effects. Table 11–8 lists some of these side effects.

Considerations for Organ Transplantation

Transplantation services often require psychiatric evalution as part of the screening process. Suggested criteria are shown in Table 11–9.

Other Issues Commonly Seen in Psychiatric Consultation

Pseudoseizures

The following are clues to a diagnosis of pseudoseizures (Cummings and Trimble 2002):

- Normal EEG (ictal or interictal) and frequent seizures

TABLE 11–8.   Selected cardiac side effects of psychotropic drugs

DRUG	CARDIAC SIDE EFFECTS
Lithium	Sinus node dysfunction and arrest
Selective serotonin reuptake inhibitor	Slowing of heart rate; occasional sinus bradycardia or sinus arrest
Tricyclic antidepressant	Orthostatic hypotension; atrioventricular conduction disturbance; type IA antiarrhythmic effect; proarrhythmia in overdose and in setting of ischemia
Monoamine oxidase inhibitor	Orthostatic hypotension
Phenothiazines	Orthostatic hypotension; QT interval prolongation; rare instances of torsades de pointes
Second-generation antipsychotics	Variable; QT interval prolongation
Carbamazepine	Type IA antiarrhythmic effects; atrioventricular block
Cholinesterase inhibitors	Decreased heart rate

- Status epilepticus (rare), especially with normal ictal or interictal EEG
- Past psychiatric history, especially personality disorders
- Paramedical professions
- Variability of phenomenology, multiple seizure descriptions
- Failure to respond to conventional antiepileptic drugs with some of the features listed above
- Pelvic thrusting seen during the attack (very rarely seen with frontal seizures)
- Crying and emotional displays after the attack

Psychological Factors Influencing Drug Refusal

Simon and Shuman (2007) listed the following psychological factors influencing drug refusal:

- Transference and countertransference issues

TABLE 11–9. Biopsychosocial screening criteria for solid organ transplantation

---

Absolute contraindications

- Active substance abuse
- Psychosis significantly limiting informed consent or compliance
- Refusal of transplant and/or active suicidal ideation
- Factitious disorder with physical symptoms
- Noncompliance with the transplant system
- Unwillingness to participate in necessary psychoeducational and psychiatric treatment

Relative contraindications

- Dementia or other persistent cerebral dysfunction, if unable to arrange adequate psychosocial resources to supervise compliance or if dysfunction known to correlate with high risk of adverse posttransplant neuropsychiatric outcome (e.g., alcohol dementia, frontal lobe syndromes)
- Treatment-refractory psychiatric illness, such as intractable, life-threatening mood disorder, schizophrenia, eating disorder, character disorder

---

Source. Adapted from Skotzko and Strouse 2002.

- Fears about taking medications
- Prior adverse reactions to medications
- Hospital staff conflicts
- Influence of family and friends
- Nonadherence as a power struggle
- Primary and secondary gain from disabling symptoms
- Denial of illness

Treating Difficult Patients

A psychiatrist may be called because a patient is causing difficulties for the staff, including being excessively demanding or critical or causing discord among the medical staff. Frequently this type of patient sees some staff members as "all good" and others as "all bad," a defense mechanism known as splitting. Splitting may cause significant discord among the staff. In these cases, the psychiatrist should help the staff understand the situation, set firm boundaries with the patient, and encourage the staff to meet with the patient together.

References

American Psychiatric Association: Diagnostic and Statistical Manual of Mental Disorders, 4th Edition, Text Revision. Washington, DC, American Psychiatric Association, 2000

American Psychiatric Association: Quick Reference to the American Psychiatric Association Practice Guidelines for the Treatment of Psychiatric Disorders: Compendium 2006. Washington, DC, American Psychiatric Publishing, 2006

Bronheim HE, Fulop G, Kunkel EJ, et al: Practice guidelines for psychiatric consultation in the general medical setting. Psychosomatics 39:S8–S30, 1998

Cohen LM, Tessier EG, Germain MJ, et al: Update on psychotropic medication use in renal disease. Psychosomatics 45:34–48, 2004

Crone CC, Gabriel GM, DiMartini A: An overview of psychiatric issues in liver disease for the consultation-liaison psychiatrist. Psychosomatics 47:188–205, 2006

Cummings JL, Trimble MR: Concise Guide to Neuropsychiatry and Behavioral Neurology, 2nd Edition. Washington, DC, American Psychiatric Publishing, 2002

Hilty DM, Seritan AL, Bourgeois JA, et al: Delirium due to a general medical condition, delirium due to multiple etiologies, and delirium not otherwise specified, in Gabbard's Treatments of Psychiatric Disorders, Fourth Edition. Edited by Gabbard GO. Washington, DC, American Psychiatric Publishing, 2007, pp 145–158

Sharpe MC, O'Mally PG : Chronic fatigue and fibromyalgia syndromes, in Essentials of Psychosomatic Medicine. Edited by Levenson JL. Washington, DC, American Psychiatric Publishing, 2007, pp 153–180

Simon RI, Shuman DW: Clinical Manual of Psychiatry and Law. Washington, DC, American Psychiatric Publishing, 2007

Skotzko CE, Strouse TB: Solid organ transplantation, in The American Psychiatric Publishing Textbook of Consultation-Liaison Psychiatry: Psychiatry in the Medically Ill, 2nd Edition. Edited by Wise MG, Rundell JR. Washington, DC, American Psychiatric Publishing, 2002, pp 623–655

Turjanski N, Lloyd GG: Psychiatric side-effects of medication: recent developments. Advances in Psychiatric Treatment 11:58–70, 2005

Williams ER, Shepherd SM: Medical clearance of psychiatric patients. Emerg Med Clin North Am 18:185–198, 2000

Wolfe F: Fibromyalgia. Rheum Dis Clin North Am 16:681–698, 1990

12

Emergency Psychiatry

This chapter contains information on psychiatric emergencies, regardless of setting, and evaluation and treatment tips for the psychiatric emergency room or department setting.

Psychiatric Emergencies

The Unconscious Psychiatric Patient

Figure 12–1 illustrates the management of the unconscious psychiatric patient.

The Potentially Violent Patient

The duty to warn third-party nonpatients of potential violent acts by patients has wide variability from state to state and is rooted in the 1976 decision of the Supreme Court of California in the *Tarasoff v. Regents of the University of California* case. About half of the states have enacted statutes pertaining to the duty of psychiatrists to warn potential victims and contain a provision for immunity for disclosure. As described by Kachigian and Felthous (2004), *duty to warn* rules generally apply in the case of foreseeable violence, foreseeable victim, identifiable victim, and specific time frame.

Dermatological Emergencies

Figure 12–2 presents an algorithm for a drug-related skin eruption. The psychiatric drugs that most commonly cause rash are lamotrigine, carbamazepine, and oxcarbazepine.

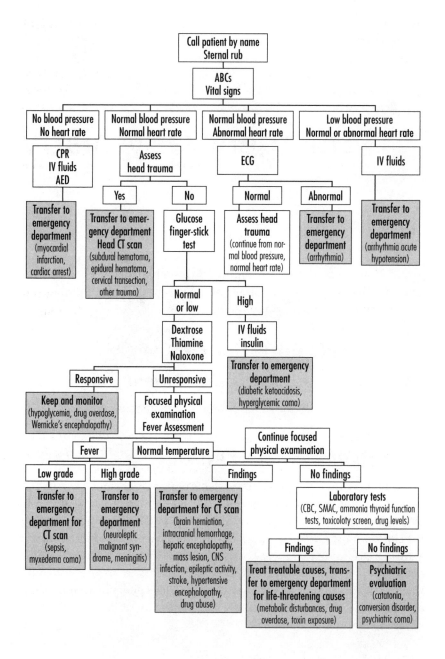

FIGURE 12–1. Management of the unconscious psychiatric patient (*opposite*).

ABCs=airway, breathing, circulation; AED=automatic external defibrillator; CBC=complete blood cell count; CNS=central nervous system; CPR=cardiopulmonary resuscitation; CT=computed tomography; ECG=electrocardiogram; EEG=electroencephalogram; IV=intravenous; SMAC=chemistry panel.

Source. Reprinted from Leibowitz S, Suarez RE: "The unresponsive psychiatric patient," in *Handbook of Medicine in Psychiatry.* Edited by Manu P, Suarez RE, Barnett BJ. Washington, DC, American Psychiatric Publishing, 2006. Used with permission.

Stevens-Johnson syndrome is a severe systemic disorder that starts with an erythematous rash 1–3 weeks after starting a medication. Characteristic symptoms include target lesions and blisters especially of the mucosal membranes, accompanied by fever and malaise.

Toxic epidermal necrolysis is similar to Stevens-Johnson syndrome but occurs within days of drug initiation, and there are no target lesions.

Serotonin Syndrome (Serotonin Toxicity)

SYMPTOMS

Serotonin syndrome is a rare condition resulting from the combination of serotonergic agents that leads to excess central nervous system serotonin. The syndrome may be fatal. The symptoms of serotonin syndrome fall into three main categories: neuromuscular excitation, autonomic effects, and mental status changes (Isbister et al. 2007).

Neuromuscular excitation

- Generalized hyperreflexia, especially in lower limbs; this symptom is key to differentiate serotonin syndrome from other conditions
- Ocular clonus or nondirectional nystagmus
- Myoclonus (often spontaneous, especially in ankle)
- Shivering
- Tremor
- Hypertonia/rigidity

Autonomic effects

- Hyperthermia (severe if body temperature is >38.4°C)
- Tachycardia

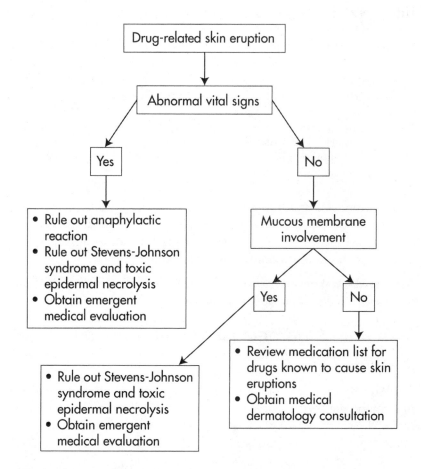

FIGURE 12–2.   Algorithm for drug-related skin eruption.

Source.   Reprinted from Valassis SA: "The unresponsive psychiatric patient," in *Handbook of Medicine in Psychiatry.* Edited by Manu P, Suarez RE, Barnett BJ. Washington, DC, American Psychiatric Publishing, 2006. Used with permission.

- Diaphoresis
- Flushing
- Mydriasis

Mental status changes
- Agitation
- Hypomania
- Anxiety

DRUGS MOST LIKELY TO CAUSE SEROTONIN SYNDROME

- Drugs most likely to cause serotonin syndrome include monoamine oxidase inhibitors (MAOIs) and any other serotonin agonists, such as selective serotonin reuptake inhibitors (SSRIs) and meperidine. Serotonin syndrome with SSRIs is potentially lethal.
- A less severe serotonin syndrome may occur when combining serotonergic drugs that do not include MAOIs, such as SSRIs plus tryptophan or SSRIs plus fenfluramine.

TREATMENT OF SEROTONIN SYNDROME

The treatment of serotonin toxicity includes the following (see also Chapter 14, "Pharmacotherapy"):

- Cessation of serotonergic medication;
- Supportive treatment, including maintaining airway, breathing, and circulation; and
- Passive and active cooling of the patient.

Acute Dystonic Reaction

Acute dystonic reaction may be seen with high-potency conventional antipsychotics and can include spasms of the neck, uncontrolled lateral eye movements (oculogyric crisis), and laryngospasm (sudden and uncontrollable closure of the larynx), which may be life-threatening. Treatment of acute dystonic reaction includes intravenous or intramuscular administration of an anticholinergic agent (e.g., Benadryl [diphenhydramine], Cogentin [benztropine mesylate]).

Lithium Toxicity

SIGNS AND SYMPTOMS

The signs and symptoms of lithium toxicity are summarized in Table 12–1.

TREATMENT

- Discontinue lithium.
- Hydrate patient.
- Perform a complete physical examination, including mental status examination.

TABLE 12–1.　Sign and symptoms of lithium toxicity

Mild to moderate (lithium level 1.5–2.0 mEq/L)

Vomiting

Abdominal pain

Dryness of mouth

Ataxia

Dizziness

Slurred speech

Nystagmus

Lethargy or excitement

Muscle weakness

Intention tremor

Moderate to severe (lithium level 2.1–2.5 mEq/L)

Anorexia

Persistent nausea or vomiting

Blurred vision

Muscle fasciculations

Clonic limb movements

Hyperactive deep tendon reflexes

Choreoathetoid movements

Convulsions

Delirium

Syncope

Electroencephalogram changes

Stupor

Coma

Circulatory failure

Severe intoxication (lithium level >2.5 mEq/L)

Generalized convulsions

Oliguria and renal failure

Death

Source.　Reprinted from Marangell LB, Martinez JM: *Concise Guide to Psychopharmacology, 2nd Edition.* Washington, DC, American Psychiatric Publishing, 2006. Used with permission.

- Check serum electrolytes and lithium levels, and perform electrocardiogram.
- For acute ingestion, use induced emesis, gastric lavage, or activated charcoal.
- Administer hemodialysis for levels greater than 4.0 mEq/L.

Anticholinergic Intoxication

Table 12–2 lists the peripheral signs and central symptoms of anticholinergic intoxication.

The Psychiatric Emergency Department

Psychiatric patients also develop medical illnesses; therefore, care must be taken when ruling out medical conditions. It is unfortunate, but often true, that any symptom in a patient with a known psychiatric disorder is attributed to the psychiatric disorder. Be especially vigilant of patients whose presentation is atypical and if there is an abrupt change or fluctuations in mental status.

- All patients in the psychiatric emergency room should have a urine drug screen.
- Patients who are an imminent threat to themselves or others or who are unable to meet their basic needs may be committed involuntarily to a psychiatric facility. Procedures vary by state, but all

TABLE 12–2. Symptoms of anticholinergic intoxication

PERIPHERAL SIGNS	CENTRAL SYMPTOMS
Mydriasis	Visual hallucinations
Tachycardia	Drowsiness
Hyperthermia	Distortion of body image
Decreased salivation	Amnesia
Dryness of skin and mucous membranes	Heat stroke (from hyperthermia at high environmental temperatures)
Facial flushing	
Difficulty urinating	

typically allow for detention for evaluation and treatment. Even in committed patients, involuntary medication is not allowed except in an acute emergency or if specifically authorized by the court.

- Do not discharge an intoxicated patient, and do not give a new psychiatric diagnosis to intoxicated patients. Ensure patient safety, watch for withdrawal, and reevaluate when the patient is sober.
- For all patients, document disposition and its rationale.

Table 12–3 presents a triage checklist for patients presenting to an emergency department with psychiatric problems.

The following information should be ascertained in a *psychosocial evaluation* (Rosenberg and Sulkowicz 2002):

- Availability of a support system and the patient's capacity to use it
- Dangerousness of a patient to self and others
- Psychiatric history and current psychiatric status
- Patient's previous methods of coping with similar stressors
- Ability to conduct self-care measures
- Motivation and capacity to participate in the treatment process
- Requests of patient and family

References

Currier GW, Allen MH, Serper MR, et al: Medical, psychiatric, and cognitive assessment in the psychiatric emergency service, in Emergency Psychiatry. Edited by Allen MH. Washington, DC, American Psychiatric Publishing, 2002, pp 35–68

Isbister GK, Buckley NA, Whyte IM: Serotonin toxicity: a practical approach to diagnosis and treatment. Med J Aust 187:361–365, 2007

Kachigian C, Felthous AR: Court responses to Tarasoff statutes. J Am Acad Psychiatry Law 32:263–273, 2004

Rosenberg RC, Sulkowicz KJ: Psychosocial interventions in the psychiatric emergency service, in Emergency Psychiatry. Edited by Allen MH. Washington, DC, American Psychiatric Publishing, 2002, pp 151–178

TABLE 12–3. Triage checklist for patients presenting to an emergency department with psychiatric problems

Identifying problem

Observe the patient's behavior.

Have the patient describe the presenting problem.

Gather data from collateral contacts.

Check vital signs.

Look for indications of physical illness.

Check current medications.

Ascertain medical and psychiatric histories.

Assessing seriousness of problem

Determine whether the patient is at risk to self or others.

Determine whether the patient presents an escape risk.

Consider whether the patient's symptoms may be due to a medical problem.

Immediate nursing care measures

Assess how long the patient can wait for further evaluation.

Prepare the environment for the patient to wait safely (e.g., remove potentially dangerous objects).

Determine what measures are needed to prevent an immediate medical emergency.

Source. Reprinted from Currier GW, Allen MH, Serper MR, et al: "Medical, Psychiatric, and Cognitive Assessment in the Psychiatric Emergency Service," in *Emergency Psychiatry*. Edited by Allen MH. Washington, DC, American Psychiatric Publishing, 2002. Used with permission.

13

Child and Adolescent Psychiatry

Developmental Milestones and Theories

Figure 13–1 summarizes the major developmental theories regarding children from birth to age 5 years. The American Academy of Pediatrics (2004) lists the following developmental milestones:

- By age 3 months
    - Brings hand to mouth
    - Is able to hold objects
    - Smiles at sound of parent's voice
    - Begins to babble
    - Imitates some movements and sounds
    - Follows moving objects with eyes
    - Watches faces intently

- By age 7 months
    - Sits with and then without support of hands
    - Transfers objects from hand to hand
    - Ability to track objects visually improves
    - Responds to own name
    - Responds to sounds by making sounds

- Uses voice to express joy and displeasure
- Enjoys social play (like peekaboo)

- By age 12 months
  - Gets to sitting position without assistance
  - Walks holding on to furniture
  - Uses pincer grasp (e.g., can pick up a Cheerio)
  - Responds to simple verbal requests
  - Says "dada" and "mama"
  - Babbles with inflection
  - Looks at correct picture when the image is named
  - Shy or anxious with strangers
  - Cries when mother or father leaves
  - Repeats sounds or gestures for attention
  - Imitates gestures (e.g., waving)

- By age 2 years
  - Walks alone using heel-toe walking pattern
  - Begins to run
  - Might use one hand more frequently than another
  - Scribbles spontaneously
  - Speaks at least 15 words (by 18 months)
  - Uses two- to four-word sentences
  - Follows simple instructions
  - Recognizes names of familiar people, objects, and body parts
  - Imitates behavior of others
  - Exhibits increasing separation anxiety toward 18 months, which fades by age 2 years
  - Demonstrates increasing independence
  - Begins to show defiant behavior

- By ages 3–4 years
  - Hops and stands on one foot for up to 5 seconds
  - Throws ball over head
  - Draws a person with two to four body parts
  - Uses scissors
  - Tells stories

- – Follows three-part commands
- – Engages in fantasy play
- – Cooperates with other children
- – Dresses and undresses with assistance
- – Negotiates solutions to conflict
- – Imagines that objects may be "monsters"
- – Views self as whole person involving body, mind, and feelings

- By ages 4–5 years
  - – Swings, climbs, hops
  - – Able to dress and undress unassisted
  - – Cares for own toilet needs
  - – Can count 10 or more objects
  - – Correctly names at least four colors
  - – Better understands the concept of time
  - – Wants to please friends
  - – Is more likely to agree to rules
  - – Is able to distinguish fantasy from reality
  - – Is sometimes demanding and sometimes eagerly cooperative
  - – Is aware of sexuality
  - – Shows more independence

Pervasive Developmental Disorders

Pervasive developmental disorders (PDDs) are disorders beginning in early childhood; they include autistic disorder and Asperger's disorder. The prevalence of these two disorders among children and adolescents in the U.S. population is estimated to be 4/10,000 and 0.26/1,000, respectively (Table 13–1).

Pervasive developmental disorders are marked by severe impairment in development resulting in three key impairments: social interactions, communication, and interests.

	Birth	2-3 months	4-5 months	7-9 months	10-12 months	15-18 months	20-24 months	30-36 months	48 months	60 months
Freud/ Abraham		ORAL PHASE				ANAL PHASE		PHALLIC PHASE	OEDIPAL PHASE	
		Passive		Aggressive		Retentive				
		Autoerotism	Primary narcissism							
M. Klein			PARANOID-SCHIZOID POSITION	DEPRESSIVE POSITION						
Erikson			BASIC TRUST VS. MISTRUST			AUTONOMY VS. SHAME AND DOUBT		INITIATIVE VS. GUILT	INDUSTRY VS. INFERIORITY	
Mahler		NORMAL AUTISM	SYMBIOSIS	DIFFERENTIATION		PRACTICING	RAPPROCHEMENT		ROAD TO OBJECT CONSTANCY	
Kernberg Masterson Rinsley		"Passive splitting"		"Active splitting"					Integration	
Defenses				Splitting hierarchy of defenses			. . . . Repression hierarchy of defenses			
Diagnoses	Autism		Childhood schizophrenia			Affective disorders	Borderline states (Narcissism)		Narcissistic states	Neurosis
			Process schizophrenia							

"Passive splitting"

Good	Bad
Inside-outside (Selfobject)	Inside-outside (Selfobject)

"Active splitting"

Good	Bad
Self Object	Self Object

Integration

Good	Bad
Good and bad	Good and bad

FIGURE 13–1. Theories of development.

This figure is an approximate display of each listed author's developmental scheme for comparison with other authors' schemes. The phases shown do not have exact correlation with age (i.e., this figure is not to be read in columns). The phases overlap, and neighboring phases may coexist. The theories of each author are not presented as exact equivalents of the similar-age stages of other authors. The diagnoses listed at the bottom are those that some developmental theorists believe match essential developmental fixations and arrests with future child and adult psychopathology.

Source. Reprinted from Marmer SS: "Theories of the Mind and Psychopathology," in *The American Psychiatric Publishing Textbook of Clinical Psychiatry, 4th Edition.* Edited by Hales RE, Yudofsky SC. Washington, DC, American Psychiatric Publishing, 2003. Used with permission.

TABLE 13–1. Prevalence estimates of selected disorders among children and adolescents in the U.S. population

DISORDER	PREVALENCE ESTIMATE
Autistic disorder	4/10,000
Asperger's disorder	0.26/1,000
ADHD	3%–5%
Conduct disorder	1.5%–3.4%
Oppositional defiant disorder	3%–10%
Tourette's disorder	1/1,000 (boys)
	1/10,000 (girls)
Mental retardation	1%–3%

Note. ADHD=attention-deficit/hyperactivity disorder.
Source. Data from Dulcan and Martini 2003.

Autistic Disorder

Table 13–2 presents the DSM-IV-TR (American Psychiatric Association 2000) diagnostic criteria for autistic disorder.

- Early diagnosis and intervention will improve outcomes.
- The mean age at which parents first become concerned about a child with autism is 19.1 months.
- The mean age at which treatment is sought is 24.1 months.
- Diagnosis is often not made until after age 6 years (Scahill 2005).
- Current evidence does not support the theory that vaccines cause autism (see www.cdc.gov/ncbddd/autism/vaccines.htm).

SPEECH AND COGNITIVE DEFICITS

Among those with autistic disorder, about half will remain mute. Immediate or delayed echolalia may be the only form of communication.

Most autistic children have mental retardation, and only 20%–30% have an IQ greater than 70.

TABLE 13–2. DSM-IV-TR criteria for autistic disorder

A. A total of six (or more) items from (1), (2), and (3), with at least two from (1), and one each from (2) and (3):

   (1) qualitative impairment in social interaction, as manifested by at least two of the following:

   (a) marked impairment in the use of multiple nonverbal behaviors such as eye-to-eye gaze, facial expression, body postures, and gestures to regulate social interaction

   (b) failure to develop peer relationships appropriate to developmental level

   (c) a lack of spontaneous seeking to share enjoyment, interests, or achievements with other people (e.g., by a lack of showing, bringing, or pointing out objects of interest)

   (d) lack of social or emotional reciprocity

   (2) qualitative impairments in communication as manifested by at least one of the following:

   (a) delay in, or total lack of, the development of spoken language (not accompanied by an attempt to compensate through alternative modes of communication such as gesture or mime)

   (b) in individuals with adequate speech, marked impairment in the ability to initiate or sustain a conversation with others

   (c) stereotyped and repetitive use of language or idiosyncratic language

   (d) lack of varied, spontaneous make-believe play or social imitative play appropriate to developmental level

   (3) restricted repetitive and stereotyped patterns of behavior, interests, and activities, as manifested by at least one of the following:

   (a) encompassing preoccupation with one or more stereotyped and restricted patterns of interest that is abnormal either in intensity or focus

   (b) apparently inflexible adherence to specific, nonfunctional routines or rituals

---

TABLE 13–2.   DSM-IV-TR criteria for autistic disorder *(continued)*

    (c) stereotyped and repetitive motor mannerisms (e.g., hand or finger flapping or twisting, or complex whole-body movements)

    (d) persistent preoccupation with parts of objects

B.   Delays or abnormal functioning in at least one of the following areas, with onset prior to age 3 years: (1) social interaction, (2) language as used in social communication, or (3) symbolic or imaginative play.

C.   The disturbance is not better accounted for by Rett's disorder or childhood disintegrative disorder.

BEHAVIORAL SYMPTOMS

- Changes in a familiar environment are distressing, particularly for children who have mental retardation. They are resistant to learning new activities.
- Patients maintain rigid routines (e.g., must eat particular foods, must line up toys a certain way).
- Patients perform stereotyped, repetitive motor acts (e.g., hand clapping, finger movements near the face).
- Motor development may be within normal milestones, but they often display unusual movements such as hand flapping, body rocking, and head banging.
- Patients may become preoccupied with specific topics (e.g., state capitals, birth dates).
- Obsessions and compulsions may develop (e.g., repeatedly asking the same question, compulsively touching certain objects).
- Mood may be labile. Giggling and crying may be unexplained.
- Sleep disturbances (e.g., difficulty falling asleep, prolonged night wakening) are common, particularly before age 8 years (Tsai 2004).

SOCIAL IMPAIRMENTS BY DEVELOPMENTAL LEVEL

Infancy

- Avoids eye contact
- Screams and cries to get needs met

- Shows little interest in the human voice
- Fails to posture to be picked up (arms raised)
- Shows little facial responsiveness
- Parents may suspect that child is deaf

Early childhood

- Continues to avoid eye contact
- Fails to seek out peer interactions
- May take parent by hand to get needs met but without appropriate facial expression
- Fails to appreciate the feelings and thoughts of others
- Does not imitate behavior
- May passively allow contact (such as sitting in parent's lap)
- Does not show age-appropriate stranger anxiety
- Does not look to parent for comfort
- Prefers solitary play and treats others as objects in play

Later childhood

- Lacks skills to initiate and maintain friendship
- May become passively involved in activities with peers
- Seldom initiates social interactions
- May develop attachment with parents or other family members
- Humor or expressions may be confusing
- May say things that are socially inappropriate
- May show extreme emotions of joy, fear, or anger but does not use facial expressions in ordinary interactions; appears wooden

ASSESSMENT

The following assessment tools may be used in the diagnosis and evaluation of autistic disorder (Scahill 2005):

- Behavioral screening tools
  - Autism Behavior Checklist (ABC)
  - Checklist of Autism in Toddlers (CHAT)
  - Childhood Autism Rating Scales (CARS)

- Physical examination
- Developmental, medical, and family history
- IQ testing
- Genetic testing
- Lead screening (if mental retardation is present)
    - Metabolic testing (with neurological deficits or regression)
    - Magnetic resonance imaging (with neurological deficits or regression)
    - Occupational therapy evaluation (with hypotonia or poor coordination)

DIFFERENTIAL DIAGNOSIS

- Regression in normal development (regression is neither as severe nor as prolonged as in autistic disorder)
- Rett's disorder (occurs only in females and is marked by head growth deceleration, loss of previously acquired hand skills, and the development of an uncoordinated gait or trunk movements)
- Childhood disintegrative disorders (characterized by a pattern of developmental regression which follows at least 2 years of normal development)
- Asperger's disorder (language impairment is absent)
- Schizophrenia (onset in childhood usually develops after years of normal development)
- Selective mutism (communication impairment is limited to select situations, and the social impairment is absent)
- Obsessive-compulsive disorder (obsessive thoughts, cleaning, counting, and checking are less frequent in autism)
- Tourette's disorder
- Lead poisoning for patients with mental retardation (Scahill 2005; Tsai 2004)

TREATMENT

- The family needs education about the disorder, realistic expectations, and supportive resources. The school will be involved in assessing special education needs.
- Pharmacological treatment is based on the targeted symptoms.

- Hyperactivity and inattention: methylphenidate, clonidine, and atomoxetine
- Aggression/self-injurious behavior: antipsychotics
- Repetitive/stereotypic behavior: clomipramine, selective serotonin reuptake inhibitors

- Behavioral therapy targets maladaptive behavior. It must be setting-specific because autistic children do not easily generalize from one setting to another.

- Sensorimotor therapies are based on the speculation that children with autism may be over- or underaroused by normal levels of sensory input. These therapies include sensory integration therapy and auditory integration therapy (Tsai 2004).

- Patients may also require speech and language therapy, social skills training, and special education services and vocational training.

Asperger's Disorder

Table 13–3 presents the DSM-IV-TR diagnostic criteria for Asperger's disorder. Treatment is similar to that described in the "Autistic Disorder" section, earlier in this chapter.

DIFFERENTIAL DIAGNOSIS

- Autistic disorder (patients with Asperger's disorder do not have delayed speech)
- Oppositional defiant disorder
- Affective disorders
- Schizophrenia
- Obsessive-compulsive disorder

Attention-Deficit/Hyperactivity Disorder

Table 13–4 presents the DSM-IV-TR diagnostic criteria for attention-deficit/hyperactivity disorder (ADHD), and Table 13–5 summarizes the presentation of ADHD through the life cycle.

TABLE 13–3.   DSM-IV-TR criteria for Asperger's disorder

A.   Qualitative impairment in social interaction, as manifested by at least two of the following:

   (1)   marked impairment in the use of multiple nonverbal behaviors such as eye-to-eye gaze, facial expression, body postures, and gestures to regulate social interaction

   (2)   failure to develop peer relationships appropriate to developmental level

   (3)   a lack of spontaneous seeking to share enjoyment, interests, or achievements with other people (e.g., by a lack of showing, bringing, or pointing out objects of interest to other people)

   (4)   lack of social or emotional reciprocity

B.   Restricted repetitive and stereotyped patterns of behavior, interests, and activities, as manifested by at least one of the following:

   (1)   encompassing preoccupation with one or more stereotyped and restricted patterns of interest that is abnormal either in intensity or focus

   (2)   apparently inflexible adherence to specific, nonfunctional routines or rituals

   (3)   stereotyped and repetitive motor mannerisms (e.g., hand or finger flapping or twisting, or complex whole-body movements)

   (4)   persistent preoccupation with parts of objects

C.   The disturbance causes clinically significant impairment in social, occupational, or other important areas of functioning.

D.   There is no clinically significant general delay in language (e.g., single words used by age 2 years, communicative phrases used by age 3 years).

E.   There is no clinically significant delay in cognitive development or in the development of age-appropriate self-help skills, adaptive behavior (other than in social interaction), and curiosity about the environment in childhood.

F.   Criteria are not met for another specific pervasive developmental disorder or schizophrenia.

TABLE 13–4. DSM-IV-TR criteria for attention-deficit/
hyperactivity disorder

A. Either (1) or (2):

(1) six (or more) of the following symptoms of **inattention** have persisted for at least 6 months to a degree that is maladaptive and inconsistent with developmental level:

Inattention

(a) often fails to give close attention to details or makes careless mistakes in schoolwork, work, or other activities

(b) often has difficulty sustaining attention in tasks or play activities

(c) often does not seem to listen when spoken to directly

(d) often does not follow through on instructions and fails to finish schoolwork, chores, or duties in the workplace (not due to oppositional behavior or failure to understand instructions)

(e) often has difficulty organizing tasks and activities

(f) often avoids, dislikes, or is reluctant to engage in tasks that require sustained mental effort (such as schoolwork or homework)

(g) often loses things necessary for tasks or activities (e.g., toys, school assignments, pencils, books, or tools)

(h) is often easily distracted by extraneous stimuli

(i) is often forgetful in daily activities

(2) six (or more) of the following symptoms of **hyperactivity-impulsivity** have persisted for at least 6 months to a degree that is maladaptive and inconsistent with developmental level:

Hyperactivity

(a) often fidgets with hands or feet or squirms in seat

(b) often leaves seat in classroom or in other situations in which remaining seated is expected

(c) often runs about or climbs excessively in situations in which it is inappropriate (in adolescents or adults, may be limited to subjective feelings of restlessness)

TABLE 13–4.   DSM-IV-TR criteria for attention-deficit/
hyperactivity disorder *(continued)*

(d) often has difficulty playing or engaging in leisure activities quietly

(e) is often "on the go" or often acts as if "driven by a motor"

(f) often talks excessively

Impulsivity

(g) often blurts out answers before questions have been completed

(h) often has difficulty awaiting turn

(i) often interrupts or intrudes on others (e.g., butts into conversations or games)

B. Some hyperactive-impulsive or inattentive symptoms that caused impairment were present before age 7 years.

C. Some impairment from the symptoms is present in two or more settings (e.g., at school [or work] and at home).

D. There must be clear evidence of clinically significant impairment in social, academic, or occupational functioning.

E. The symptoms do not occur exclusively during the course of a pervasive developmental disorder, schizophrenia, or other psychotic disorder and are not better accounted for by another mental disorder (e.g., mood disorder, anxiety disorder, dissociative disorder, or a personality disorder).

Code based on type:

314.01   Attention-deficit/hyperactivity disorder, combined type: if both criteria A1 and A2 are met for the past 6 months

314.00   Attention-deficit/hyperactivity disorder, predominantly inattentive type: if criterion A1 is met but criterion A2 is not met for the past 6 months

314.01   Attention-deficit/hyperactivity disorder, predominantly hyperactive-impulsive type: if criterion A2 is met but criterion A1 is not met for the past 6 months

Coding note: For individuals (especially adolescents and adults) who currently have symptoms that no longer meet full criteria, "in partial remission" should be specified.

TABLE 13–5. Presentation of attention-deficit/hyperactivity disorder (ADHD) through the life cycle

DEVELOPMENTAL STAGE	CHARACTERISTICS OF ADHD	COMMENTS
Infancy	Frequent crying, difficult to soothe, sleep disturbances, feeding difficulties	May cry to extent that it interferes with nutritional intake, may be excessively drowsy or unresponsive or sleep poorly because of overreactivity and restlessness
Preschool	Motor restlessness, insatiable curiosity, vigorous and sometimes destructive play, demanding of parental attention, excessive temper tantrums, difficulty completing developmental tasks	Often difficult to distinguish from normal behaviors in children this age; climbs on and gets into things constantly; often accidentally breaks toys and household items; accidental injuries are common
School-age	Easily distracted; engages in "off-task" activities; acts as "class clown"; displays aggression; has social deficits; has difficulty waiting turn, following rules, and losing gracefully; frequently becomes overly excited	May call out in class inappropriately; fidgets excessively; homework is messy and disorganized; academic performance and peer relationships are affected, and failures in these areas lead to poor self-esteem and depression

TABLE 13–5. Presentation of attention-deficit/hyperactivity disorder (ADHD) through the life cycle *(continued)*

DEVELOPMENTAL STAGE	CHARACTERISTICS OF ADHD	COMMENTS
Adolescence	Excessive motor activity tends to decrease, fidgetiness and inner restlessness may continue; family conflict, anger and emotional lability, difficulty with authority, poor peer relationships, poor self-esteem, lethargy and poor self-esteem, driving mishaps	Impulsive symptoms may lead to breaking rules and conflict with authorities
Adult	Difficulty concentrating and performing sedentary tasks, disorganization, forgetfulness, losing things, failure to plan, trouble starting and finishing tasks, misjudging time, being absentminded	May have employment difficulties, especially at desk jobs; higher incidence of antisocial acts and arrests than general population

Source. Adapted from Popper et al. 2003.

Symptom scales and other assessments may be useful to supplement clinical information (Waslick and Greenhill 2004):

- Child Behavior Checklist (CBCL)
- Conners' Teacher Rating Scale
- Continuous Performance Test

Differential Diagnosis

- Language disorders
- Sydenham chorea
- Tourette's disorder
- Conduct disorder
- Mental retardation

Treatment

PHARMACOLOGY

- Stimulants of the nonstimulant norepinephrine reuptake inhibitor atomoxetine are the primary treatments. Use of stimulants results in decreased appetite and may raise the risk of tics in patients with a personal or family history of tic disorder. Growth needs to be monitored. Use of stimulants may reduce the risk for substance use disorder.
- Tricyclic antidepressants are rarely used.
- Other medications sometimes used in ADHD include bupropion, modafinil, and α_2-adrenergic agonists.

The use of these medications is discussed in more detail in Chapter 14, "Pharmacotherapy."

PSYCHOSOCIAL INTERVENTIONS

Psychosocial interventions in ADHD include behavioral modification and cognitive-behavioral therapy.

Conduct Disorder and Oppositional Defiant Disorder

Tables 13–6 and 13–7 present the DSM-IV-TR diagnostic criteria for conduct disorder and oppositional defiant disorder, respectively.

Differential Diagnosis

- ADHD
- Learning disabilities
- Mood disorder
- Dissociative disorder
- Seizures or other central nervous system dysfunction

Treatment

Skills training and pharmacotherapy are used in the treatment of conduct disorder and oppositional defiant disorder (Hendren and Mullen 2004), specifically:

- Problem-solving skills training (e.g., anger management, problem solving, communication skills)
- Family treatments (e.g., parent management training, teaching behavioral techniques, interpersonal problem solving)
- Social skills training
- Pharmacotherapy to treat aggression or comorbid condition

TABLE 13–6. DSM-IV-TR criteria for conduct disorder

A. A repetitive and persistent pattern of behavior in which the basic rights of others or major age-appropriate societal norms or rules are violated, as manifested by the presence of three (or more) of the following criteria in the past 12 months, with at least one criterion present in the past 6 months:

Aggression to people and animals

(1) often bullies, threatens, or intimidates others

(2) often initiates physical fights

(3) has used a weapon that can cause serious physical harm to others (e.g., a bat, brick, broken bottle, knife, gun)

(4) has been physically cruel to people

(5) has been physically cruel to animals

(6) has stolen while confronting a victim (e.g., mugging, purse snatching, extortion, armed robbery)

(7) has forced someone into sexual activity

Destruction of property

(8) has deliberately engaged in fire setting with the intention of causing serious damage

(9) has deliberately destroyed others' property (other than by fire setting)

Deceitfulness or theft

(10) has broken into someone else's house, building, or car

(11) often lies to obtain goods or favors or to avoid obligations (i.e., "cons" others)

(12) has stolen items of nontrivial value without confronting a victim (e.g., shoplifting, but without breaking and entering; forgery)

Serious violations of rules

(13) often stays out at night despite parental prohibitions, beginning before age 13 years

(14) has run away from home overnight at least twice while living in parental or parental surrogate home (or once without returning for a lengthy period)

(15) is often truant from school, beginning before age 13 years

---

TABLE 13–6.   DSM-IV-TR criteria for conduct disorder *(continued)*

B.   The disturbance in behavior causes clinically significant impairment in social, academic, or occupational functioning.

C.   If the individual is age 18 years or older, criteria are not met for antisocial personality disorder.

Code based on age at onset:

> **312.81   Conduct disorder, childhood-onset type:**   onset of at least one criterion characteristic of conduct disorder prior to age 10 years
>
> **312.82   Conduct disorder, adolescent-onset type:**   absence of any criteria characteristic of conduct disorder prior to age 10 years
>
> **312.89   Conduct disorder, unspecified onset:**   age at onset is not known

Specify severity:

> **Mild:**   few if any conduct problems in excess of those required to make the diagnosis **and** conduct problems cause only minor harm to others
>
> **Moderate:**   number of conduct problems and effect on others intermediate between "mild" and "severe"
>
> **Severe:**   many conduct problems in excess of those required to make the diagnosis **or** conduct problems cause considerable harm to others

---

Tourette's Disorder

Table 13–8 presents the DSM-IV-TR diagnostic criteria for Tourette's disorder.

Differential Diagnosis

The differential diagnosis includes the following conditions (King and Leckman 2004):

- Other dyskinesias (e.g., myoclonus, choreoathetosis, akathisia, and tardive dyskinesias)
- Obsessive-compulsive disorder

TABLE 13–7. DSM-IV-TR criteria for oppositional defiant disorder

---

A. A pattern of negativistic, hostile, and defiant behavior lasting at least 6 months, during which four (or more) of the following are present:

   (1) often loses temper

   (2) often argues with adults

   (3) often actively defies or refuses to comply with adults' requests or rules

   (4) often deliberately annoys people

   (5) often blames others for his or her mistakes or misbehavior

   (6) is often touchy or easily annoyed by others

   (7) is often angry and resentful

   (8) is often spiteful or vindictive

   Note: Consider a criterion met only if the behavior occurs more frequently than is typically observed in individuals of comparable age and developmental level.

B. The disturbance in behavior causes clinically significant impairment in social, academic, or occupational functioning.

C. The behaviors do not occur exclusively during the course of a psychotic or mood disorder.

D. Criteria are not met for conduct disorder, and, if the individual is age 18 years or older, criteria are not met for antisocial personality disorder.

- Psychogenic tics
- Stereotypes, as in PDD

Treatment

- Pharmacotherapy: α-adrenergic agents, while more benign, are less potent. Antipsychotics are typical first-line pharmacotherapy.
- Cognitive-behavioral therapy (e.g., exposure and response prevention)
- Habit reversal techniques
- Treatment of comorbid conditions such as ADHD and obsessive-compulsive disorder

---

TABLE 13–8.   DSM-IV-TR criteria for Tourette's disorder

A. Both multiple motor and one or more vocal tics have been present at some time during the illness, although not necessarily concurrently. (A *tic* is a sudden, rapid, recurrent, nonrhythmic, stereotyped motor movement or vocalization.)

B. The tics occur many times a day (usually in bouts) nearly every day or intermittently throughout a period of more than 1 year, and during this period there was never a tic-free period of more than 3 consecutive months.

C. The onset is before age 18 years.

D. The disturbance is not due to the direct physiological effects of a substance (e.g., stimulants) or a general medical condition (e.g., Huntington's disease or postviral encephalitis).

Mental Retardation

Table 13–9 presents the DSM-IV-TR diagnostic criteria for mental retardation.

Levels of Mental Retardation

- Mild: IQ 50–55 to 70
- Moderate: IQ 35–40 to 50–55
- Severe: IQ 20–25 to 35–40
- Profound: IQ below 20

Assessment

- Physical examination
- Chromosomal analysis
- Metabolic screening
- Computed tomography or magnetic resonance imaging

Differential Diagnosis

- Learning disability
- Communication disorder
- PDD

TABLE 13–9. **DSM-IV-TR criteria for mental retardation**

A. Significantly subaverage intellectual functioning: an IQ of approximately 70 or below on an individually administered IQ test (for infants, a clinical judgment of significantly subaverage intellectual functioning).

B. Concurrent deficits or impairments in present adaptive functioning (i.e., the person's effectiveness in meeting the standards expected for his or her age by his or her cultural group) in at least two of the following areas: communication, self-care, home living, social/ interpersonal skills, use of community resources, self-direction, functional academic skills, work, leisure, health, and safety.

C. The onset is before age 18 years.

Code based on degree of severity reflecting level of intellectual impairment:

317 **Mild mental retardation:** IQ level 50–55 to approx. 70

318.0 **Moderate mental retardation:** IQ level 35–40 to 50–55

318.1 **Severe mental retardation:** IQ level 20–25 to 35–40

318.2 **Profound mental retardation:** IQ level below 20 or 25

319 **Mental retardation, severity unspecified:** when there is strong presumption of mental retardation but the person's intelligence is untestable by standard tests

---

Treatment

The goal of treatment is to achieve the best-possible quality of life. Treatment options include ((Szymanski and Kaplan 2004):

- Treatment directed at the underlying cause (e.g., hypothyroidism, phenylketonuria)
- Behavior modification
- Psychotherapy (based on patient's communication skills): may include modeling of real-life situation problem solving
- Family-directed intervention
- Pharmacotherapy: should be used judiciously to treat specific symptoms and to improve the quality of life. The frequency of side effects in this population may be different from that of

patients without mental retardation. For example, patients with Down syndrome may be very sensitive to anticholinergic drugs, and some medications may cause further cognitive dulling.

Major Depressive Disorder

The characteristics of child and adolescent presentation of major depressive disorder include the following (Weller et al. 2004):

- More somatic complaints
- Increased psychomotor agitation
- Increased mood-congruent hallucinations
- Increased comorbid anxiety
- Antisocial behavior
- Substance abuse
- Grouchiness
- Aggression
- Withdrawal

For more information on major depressive disorder, see Chapter 3, "Mood Disorders."

Bipolar Disorder

The characteristics of child and adolescent presentation of bipolar disorder include the following (Weller et al. 2004):

- Irritability with affective "storms" and aggressive temper outbursts
- Worsening of disruptive behavior
- Difficulty sleeping at night
- Impulsivity
- Explosive anger
- High rates of comorbidity (especially externalizing disorders)

For more information on bipolar disorder, see Chapter 3, "Mood Disorders."

References

American Academy of Pediatrics: Caring for Your Baby and Young Child: Birth to Age 5. Edited by Shelov SP, Hannemann RE. New York, Bantam Books, 2004

American Psychiatric Association: Diagnostic and Statistical Manual of Mental Disorders, 4th Edition, Text Revision. Washington, DC, American Psychiatric Association, 2000

Dulcan MK, Martini DR: Concise Guide to Child and Adolescent Psychiatry, 3rd Edition. Washington, DC, American Psychiatric Press, 2003

Hendren RL, Mullen DJ: Conduct disorder and oppositional defiant disorder, in The American Psychiatric Publishing Textbook of Child and Adolescent Psychiatry, 3rd Edition. Edited by Wiener JM, Dulcan MK. Washington, DC, American Psychiatric Publishing, 2004, pp 509–528

King RA, Leckman JF: Tic disorders, in The American Psychiatric Publishing Textbook of Child and Adolescent Psychiatry, 3rd Edition. Edited by Wiener JM, Dulcan MK. Washington, DC, American Psychiatric Publishing, 2004, pp 709–726

Popper CW, Gammon GD, West SA, et al: Disorders usually first diagnosed in infancy, childhood, or adolescence, in The American Psychiatric Publishing Textbook of Clinical Psychiatry, 4th Edition. Edited by Hales RE, Yudofsky SC. Washington, DC, American Psychiatric Publishing, 2003, pp 833–974

Scahill L: Diagnosis and evaluation of pervasive developmental disorders. J Clin Psychiatry, 66 (suppl 10):19–25, 2005

Szymanski LS, Kaplan KC: Mental retardation, in The American Psychiatric Publishing Textbook of Child and Adolescent Psychiatry, 3rd Edition. Edited by Wiener JM, Dulcan MK. Washington, DC, American Psychiatric Publishing, 2004, pp 221–260

Tsai LY: Autistic disorders, in The American Psychiatric Publishing Textbook of Child and Adolescent Psychiatry, 3rd Edition. Edited by Wiener JM, Dulcan MK. Washington, DC, American Psychiatric Publishing, 2004, pp 261–316

Waslick B, Greenhill LL: Attention deficit/hyperactivity disorder, in The American Psychiatric Publishing Textbook of Child and Adolescent Psychiatry, 3rd Edition. Edited by Wiener JM, Dulcan MK. Washington, DC, American Psychiatric Publishing, 2004, pp 485–508

Weller EG, Weller RA, Danielyan AK: Mood disorders in prepubertal children, in The American Psychiatric Publishing Textbook of Child and Adolescent Psychiatry, 3rd Edition. Edited by Wiener JM, Dulcan MK. Washington, DC, American Psychiatric Publishing, 2004, pp 411–436

14

Pharmacotherapy

Antipsychotics

- Antipsychotic medications are effective for the treatment of a variety of psychotic symptoms such as hallucinations, delusions, and thought disorders, regardless of etiology.

- The term *conventional* is used to signify older or first-generation antipsychotic drugs and to differentiate them from newer, atypical or second-generation antipsychotics. All conventional antipsychotics are equally effective when given in equivalent doses.

- Although the term *atypical antipsychotic* lacks a single consistent definition, it generally implies fewer extrapyramidal side effects (EPS), a decreased likelihood to produce hyperprolactinemia, and superior efficacy, particularly for the negative symptoms of schizophrenia.

- The efficacy and favorable neurological side-effect profiles of atypical antipsychotics have led to the recommendation for their uniform use as first-line agents—with the exception of clozapine, the use of which is restricted because of the risk of agranulocytosis (see "Clozapine" subsection later in this chapter).

Mechanisms of Action

- Underactivity of dopamine (see Table 14–1) in mesocortical pathways is thought to account for the negative symptoms of schizophrenia (e.g., anergia, apathy, lack of spontaneity).

TABLE 14–1. Common receptors in psychopharmacology

Receptor	Subtypes	Comments
Dopamine (DA)	5	D_2 is related to movement disorders. All neuroleptics bind to DA, and the antipsychotic effect of typical neuroleptics is related to the intensity of DA binding. It is abundant in striatum.
		D_1 has relevance in psychosis.
		Clozapine has relatively greater affinity for D_4.
Norepinephrine (NE)	α, β	Predominant in cortex, limbic system, and striatum
		Type α_2 is linked to depression.
Serotonin (5-HT)	At least 11	5-HT_{1A} is linked to anxiety and depression.
		5-HT_{1D} is linked to migraine.
		5-HT_2 is linked to depression, sexual function, and sleep.
		5-HT_3 is linked to nausea.
GABA	A, B	Linked to the benzodiazepine receptor
		On activation, chloride channels open.
		Inhibitory
		Abundant all over brain
		Type A linked to seizures and anxiety.

TABLE 14–1. Common receptors in psychopharmacology *(continued)*

RECEPTOR	SUBTYPES	COMMENTS
Acetylcholine	Nicotinic, muscarinic	Linked to memory and cognition; five types of muscarinic receptors now identified
Peptides	Many	Includes opiate-binding sites.
Glutamate	NMDA, AMPA	Related to seizures and memory; possible mood effects

Note. Many of these receptors have subtypes not noted here. AMPA=α-amino-3-hydroxy-5-methyl-4-isoxazole propionic acid; GABA=γ-aminobutyric acid; 5-HT=5-hydroxytryptamine; NMDA=*N*-methyl-D-aspartate.

Source. Adapted from Cummings and Trimble 2002.

- Underactivity in the frontal lobes may serve to disinhibit meso-limbic dopamine activity via a corticolimbic feedback loop. Over-activity of mesolimbic dopamine is the result, which manifests as the positive symptoms of schizophrenia (e.g., hallucinations, delusions).
- Antipsychotic medications antagonize dopamine.
- Atypical antipsychotics have other properties as well. Some of these appear to relate to antagonism of the serotonin type 2 receptor (5-HT$_2$), which is believed to account, at least in part, for the superior efficacy and more favorable side-effect profile of atypical antipsychotics.

Indications and Efficacy

- The most common indications for antipsychotic drugs are the treatment of acute psychosis and the maintenance of remission of psychotic symptoms in patients with schizophrenia. Atypicals are considered first-line agents for the treatment of schizophrenia.
- Antipsychotic drugs are indicated for the treatment of bipolar disorder.
    - All atypicals except clozapine and paliperidone have U.S. Food and Drug Administration (FDA) indication to treat acute mania.
    - Olanzapine and aripiprazole have FDA indication to treat the maintenance phase.
    - Quetiapine and the combination of olanzapine with fluoxetine have FDA indication to treat bipolar depression.
- Antipsychotic drugs are indicated for the treatment of psychotic symptoms associated with drug toxicities, delusional disorders, and nonspecific agitation.
- Low doses of antipsychotics may be effective in some patients with borderline or schizotypal personality disorders, particularly when psychotic ideation is targeted (Oldham 2005).
- Antipsychotic drugs may be used in augmentation therapy for severe obsessive-compulsive disorder (OCD).
- Tourette's disorder may be controlled with antipsychotic agents; haloperidol and pimozide are the most frequently used drugs for this disorder.

Medication Selection

- The choice of antipsychotic medication is often determined by anticipated side effects.
- Usually, atypical antipsychotics (except for clozapine) are best tolerated and are first-line agents.
- Clozapine is generally reserved for patients with refractory illness, because of the risk of agranulocytosis.
- Fluphenazine, haloperidol, and risperidone are the only antipsychotic medications currently available as long-acting injectables in the United States.

Risks, Side Effects, and Their Management

Many side effects of antipsychotic drugs as a class can be understood in terms of the drugs' receptor-blocking properties.

EXTRAPYRAMIDAL SIDE EFFECTS (EPS)

- When antipsychotics reduce dopamine activity in the nigrostriatal pathway (via dopamine receptor blockade), extrapyramidal signs and symptoms similar to those of Parkinson's disease result.
  - EPS include acute dystonic reactions, parkinsonian syndrome, akathisia, tardive dyskinesia, and neuroleptic malignant syndrome (NMS).
  - Although high-potency conventional antipsychotics are more likely to cause EPS, all first-generation antipsychotic drugs are equally likely to cause tardive dyskinesia.
  - The atypical antipsychotics cause substantially fewer EPS, which is part of the reason they are recommended as first-line agents.
  - At high doses, risperidone exhibits EPS similar to the high-potency conventional agents.

Acute dystonic reactions

- Reactions occur within hours or days of starting a high-potency conventional antipsychotic.
- Dystonic reactions are characterized by uncontrollable tightening of muscles, including spasms of the neck, back (opisthotonos), tongue, or muscles that control lateral eye movement (oculogyric crisis).

- Laryngeal involvement may compromise the airway and result in ventilatory difficulties (stridor).
- An acute dystonic reaction should be treated with intravenous or intramuscular administration of anticholinergic medication (see Table 14–2). Because antipsychotic drugs have long half-lives and durations of action, additional oral anticholinergic drugs should be prescribed for several days after an acute dystonic reaction, or longer if treatment with the antipsychotic drug is continued unchanged.

Parkinsonian syndrome

- Parkinsonian syndrome has many of the features of classic idiopathic Parkinson's disease: diminished range of facial expression (masklike facies), cogwheel rigidity, slowed movements (bradykinesia), drooling, small handwriting (micrographia), and pill-rolling tremor.
- The pathophysiology involves the presence of disproportionately less dopamine than acetylcholine in the basal ganglia.
- Onset is gradual and may not appear for weeks after antipsychotics have been administered.
- Treatment usually involves decreasing the level of acetylcholine. Amantadine, a dopaminergic drug, often effectively attenuates parkinsonian side effects without exacerbating the underlying psychotic illness.

Akathisia

- Akathisia is a subjective feeling of restlessness in the lower extremities, often manifested as an inability to sit still.
- This side effect occurs shortly after starting a conventional antipsychotic or aripiprazole.
- Treatment involves switching from a conventional antipsychotic to an atypical antipsychotic, adding a β-adrenergic-blocking drug (particularly propranolol, up to 120 mg/day), lowering the dose of aripiprazole, or switching from aripiprazole to a different atypical antipsychotic.

Tardive dyskinesia

- Tardive dyskinesia is characterized by involuntary choreoathetoid movements of the face, trunk, or extremities.

TABLE 14–2. Drugs commonly used to treat acute extrapyramidal side effects

DRUG	DRUG TYPE	USUAL DOSAGE	INDICATIONS
Amantadine (Symmetrel)	Dopaminergic agent	100 mg po bid	Parkinsonian syndrome
Benztropine (Cogentin)	Anticholinergic agent	1–2 mg po bid	Dystonia, parkinsonian syndrome
		2 mg iv[a]	Acute dystonia
Diphenhydramine (Benadryl)	Anticholinergic agent	25–50 mg po tid	Dystonia, parkinsonian syndrome
		25 mg im or iv[a]	Acute dystonia
Propranolol (Inderal)	Beta-blocker	20 mg po tid	Akathisia
		1 mg iv	
Trihexyphenidyl (Artane)	Anticholinergic agent	5–10 mg po bid	Dystonia, parkinsonian syndrome

Note. bid = twice a day; im = intramuscularly; iv = intravenously; po = orally; tid = three times a day.
[a]Follow with oral medication.

- This side effect has a cumulative incidence of 5% per year of exposure among young adults and a prevalence of 30% after 1 year of treatment with conventional antipsychotics among elderly patients.
- Clozapine seems to carry little or no risk of inducing tardive dyskinesia.
- If discontinuation of the antipsychotic drug is possible, gradual improvement of tardive dyskinesia may occur.
- Tardive dyskinesia often worsens initially with tapering of the antipsychotic dose, a phenomenon known as *withdrawal-emergent dyskinesia*. This may occur when a conventional antipsychotic is replaced with an atypical antipsychotic; it typically resolves within 6 weeks.
- There is no definitive treatment for tardive dyskinesia.
- In several small studies, α-tocopherol (vitamin E) was shown to be of some benefit; the typical dosage of vitamin E is 1,600 IU/day.

Neuroleptic malignant syndrome

- Neuroleptic malignant syndrome is potentially life-threatening.
- This side effect occurs most frequently with high-potency conventional antipsychotic drugs, but may appear during treatment with any antipsychotic agent, including atypical antipsychotics.
- Patients with NMS typically exhibit marked muscle rigidity, fever, autonomic instability, increased white blood cell count (WBC; >15,000/mm^3), increased creatine phosphokinase levels (>300 U/mL), and delirium. Muscle breakdown can lead to myoglobinuria and acute renal failure.
- Treatment includes discontinuation of the antipsychotic, administration of intravenous fluids and antipyretic agents, use of cooling blankets, and the use of dantrolene or bromocriptine.
  - Bromocriptine is given initially at 1.25–2.5 mg bid; it may be increased to 10 mg tid.
  - Dantrolene is given at a dose of 1 mg/kg by rapid intravenous push; it should be continued until the symptoms are reversed or until a maximum dose of 10 mg/kg has been given. The oral dosage is 4–8 mg/kg/day in four divided doses; this regimen should be continued until all symptoms resolve. Because the potential for hepatotoxicity is significant, dantrolene should not be given to patients with liver dysfunction.

ANTICHOLINERGIC SIDE EFFECTS

Anticholinergic side effects are categorized as peripheral or central. The most common *peripheral* side effects are dry mouth, decreased sweating, decreased bronchial secretions, blurred vision, difficulty with urination, constipation, and tachycardia. These side effects are treated with bethanechol, a cholinergic drug that does not cross the blood-brain barrier, 25–50 mg tid.

Central side effects of anticholinergic drugs include impairment in concentration, attention, and memory. These symptoms need to be distinguished from those caused by the patient's psychosis. In cases of toxicity, *anticholinergic delirium*—which includes hot, dry skin; dry mucous membranes; dilated pupils; absent bowel sounds; tachycardia; and confusion—may occur; this is a medical emergency that requires full supportive medical care. Physostigmine is an acetylcholinesterase inhibitor and may be used as a diagnostic agent if anticholinergic toxicity is suspected; it should not be used to maintain reversal of the toxicity.

ADRENERGIC SIDE EFFECTS

Antagonism of α_1-adrenergic receptors results in hypotension and dizziness.

WEIGHT GAIN

- Treatment with most atypical antipsychotics is associated with a rapid increase in body weight during the first few months of therapy.
- The rate of weight gain decreases with time, but some patients continue to gain weight even after 1 year of treatment.
- Antipsychotics associated with weight gain include risperidone, quetiapine, chlorpromazine, sertindole, thioridazine, olanzapine, and clozapine.
- The amount of weight gain is not dose dependent.

ENDOCRINE EFFECTS

- Hyperglycemia can develop independent of or secondary to weight gain; in some cases, it resolves after discontinuation of the medication.
- Patients taking clozapine and olanzapine have a higher risk of developing diabetes and have the greatest increases in total cho-

lesterol, low-density lipoprotein (LDL), and triglycerides and decreases in high-density lipoprotein (HDL) compared with patients being treated with other conventional and atypical antipsychotics.

- Aripiprazole and ziprasidone do not appear to be associated with dyslipidemia.
- Serum glucose and lipids should be checked when starting an antipsychotic and at various points throughout treatment.

SEXUAL SIDE EFFECTS

- In the pituitary and hypothalamus (the tuberoinfundibular system), dopamine is synonymous with prolactin-inhibiting factor. Blockade of dopamine here results in hyperprolactinemia.
  - Hyperprolactinemia may occur with all conventional antipsychotic medications and with risperidone.
  - Side effects mediated, at least in part, by hyperprolactinemia include gynecomastia, galactorrhea, amenorrhea, and decreased libido.

- Thioridazine may cause painful retrograde ejaculation.

OCULAR EFFECTS

- Antipsychotic drugs may cause pigmentary changes in the lens and retina.
- Pigment deposition in the lens of the eye does not affect vision.
- Pigmentary retinopathy, which can lead to irreversible blindness, has been associated with thioridazine.

CARDIAC EFFECTS

- There are several reports of sudden death attributed to thioridazine or chlorpromazine therapy in young, healthy patients.
- Thioridazine produces the greatest mean delay in QTc, followed by ziprasidone, quetiapine, olanzapine, and haloperidol.
- Pimozide may also produce significant changes in cardiac conduction as a result of its calcium channel–blocking properties. Pimozide should be discontinued if the QT interval exceeds 520 milliseconds in adults or 470 milliseconds in children; this

guideline should be considered in patients taking thioridazine and ziprasidone, but it is not mandatory in healthy patients.

- Extremely high doses of intravenous haloperidol have been administered safely in patients with cardiac disease, although rare cases of torsades de pointes have been reported at these doses.

LOWERED SEIZURE THRESHOLD

- Most antipsychotics are associated with a dose-dependent risk of a lowered seizure threshold.
- Molindone and fluphenazine have most consistently been shown to have the lowest potential for this side effect.
- Clozapine dose-dependently lowers the seizure threshold.

RISKS IN ELDERLY PATIENTS WITH DEMENTIA

- Atypical antipsychotics have been associated with an almost two-fold increased mortality when used in elderly patients with dementia.
- These medications are not approved for treatment of dementia-related psychosis, but such use is common in clinical practice (Herrmann and Lanctôt 2005).

Use of Antipsychotics in Pregnancy

- Like most other drugs, antipsychotic agents should be avoided, if possible, during pregnancy and lactation.
- The use of low-potency phenothiazine antipsychotics during the first trimester of pregnancy may increase the baseline risk of congenital anomalies by 0.4%.
- Compared with conventional antipsycotics, less is known about the risks for teratogenicity, perinatal complications, and neurobehavioral problems associated with atypical antipsychotic medications.
- Thus far, retrospective studies, case reports, and clinical observations indicate that clozapine and olanzapine are not associated with an increased teratogenic risk.
- Data related to the use of aripiprazole, quetiapine, risperidone, and ziprasidone in pregnancy are still limited.

- There is an increased risk of fetal death in psychotic mothers, so any risk of antipsychotic-induced teratogenesis must be assessed carefully and balanced against the risks involved in withholding treatment.
- The risk of developing hyperglycemia with atypical antipsychotics during pregnancy must be considered.

Atypical Antipsychotics

- Atypical antipsychotics cause fewer EPS than conventional antipsychotics.
- Clozapine and quetiapine are the least likely to cause EPS and are therefore recommended for treatment of psychosis in patients with Parkinson's disease.
- With the exception of risperidone and paliperidone, atypical antipsychotics cause substantially less hyperprolactinemia than do conventional antipsychotics.
- Weight gain is a side effect of all atypical antipsychotics except ziprasidone and aripiprazole.

CLOZAPINE (TABLET, ORAL DISINTEGRATING TABLET)

Clinical use

- Initial dosing: Start at 12.5 mg/day and quickly increase to 12.5 mg bid. Then increase as tolerated, generally in 25- or 50-mg increments every day or every other day.
- Clozapine is the only antipsychotic not associated with treatment-emergent tardive dyskinesia, and it can be used to treat patients with tardive dyskinesia.
- Clozapine is usually added to the previous antipsychotic agent in a cross-titration in which the dosage of the previous drug is tapered when a clozapine dosage of approximately 100 mg/day has been achieved. Use caution if the existing medication is a low-potency conventional antipsychotic, because of the possibility of additive α-adrenergic and anticholinergic side effects.
- The typical target dosage is 300–500 mg/day in divided doses, with a greater amount given in the evening to minimize daytime sedation.
- Serum levels should be obtained in nonresponders (350 ng/mL is associated with a higher response rate).

- The oral disintegrating tablet is bioequivalent to the oral tablet.
- Response is typically assessed after 3–6 months of treatment; if no response after 6 months, dosage may be increased to 900 mg/day.

Risks, side effects, and their management

Agranulocytosis

- Agranulocytosis is estimated to occur in 0.8% of patients treated with clozapine during the first year; peak incidence is at 3 months.
- Initial WBC must be >3,500/mm^3, and the absolute neutrophil count (ANC) must be >2,000/mm^3.
- Weekly WBC and ANC are required for the first 6 months of treatment and for 4 weeks after discontinuation of clozapine. After 6 months, monitoring is required every 2 weeks; after 12 months, monitoring is required every 4 weeks.
- If agranulocytosis develops, immediately consult a hematologist.
- Once a patient has developed agranulocytosis while taking clozapine, he or she should not be rechallenged.
- Clozapine treatment is contraindicated for patients who have myeloproliferative disorders or who are immunocompromised due to diseases such as active tuberculosis or HIV. Also, concomitant administration of medications that are associated with bone marrow suppression, such as carbamazepine, is contraindicated.

Extrapyramidal side effects

- Extrapyramidal side effects are uncommon at any dose.
- Some patients experience akathisia or hand tremors.
- There have been reports of NMS in patients medicated with clozapine alone.

Sedation

- Sedation is the most common side effect, and it is prominent early in treatment.
- Sedation generally attenuates when the dose is reduced, when tolerance to this side effect develops, or when a disproportionate amount is given at bedtime.

Cardiovascular effects

- Orthostatic hypotension and tachycardia are seen in most patients treated with clozapine.
- Cases of myocarditis and dilated cardiomyopathy have been reported (Kilian et al. 1999).
  - Myocarditis typically occurs within 3 weeks of starting clozapine, but cardiomyopathy may not be apparent for several years.
  - Although rare, treatment-emergent myocarditis and cardiomyopathy occur at a reportedly higher incidence with clozapine than with other antipsychotics.

Weight gain

Weight gain occurs in most patients treated with clozapine, with increases of 10% or more of base body weight in many patients. The weight gain is not dose related.

Hypersalivation

Hypersalivation is seen in one-third of patients treated with clozapine.

Fever

Clozapine treatment is associated with benign, transient temperature increases, usually within the first 3 weeks. The patient should be evaluated for NMS, infections, and agranulocytosis.

Seizures

Clozapine treatment is associated with a dose-dependent risk of seizures. With dosages less than 300 mg/day, there is a 1% risk of seizures; with dosages of 300–600 mg/day, there is a 2.7% risk; and with dosages greater than 600 mg/day, there is a 4.4% risk. Since patients with fairly refractory illnesses tend to receive clozapine, treatment with this medication is usually continued after a seizure, with the addition of an anticonvulsant. Carbamazepine should be avoided because of the added risk of bone marrow suppression. Valproate appears to be the safest anticonvulsant for patients taking clozapine.

Anticholinergic side effects

Dry mouth, blurred vision, constipation, and urinary retention are common early side effects of clozapine treatment.

Obsessive-compulsive disorder symptoms

Clozapine is reported to exacerbate OCD symptoms, probably because of 5-HT$_2$ antagonism. The symptoms are usually controlled with the addition of a selective serotonin reuptake inhibitor (SSRI).

Drug interactions

- Clozapine should not be combined with any drugs that can suppress the bone marrow.
- Combining clozapine with benzodiazepines (particularly in high doses) may cause respiratory arrest.
- Clozapine is metabolized by cytochrome P450 (CYP) 1A2 and, to a lesser extent, CYP 3A3/4.
  - Serum levels increase with fluvoxamine or erythromycin; this is especially important because of dose-dependent risk of seizures.
  - Serum levels decrease with phenobarbital or phenytoin and with cigarette smoking.

RISPERIDONE (TABLET, ORAL DISINTEGRATING TABLET, LIQUID)

Clinical use

- Initial dosing: Start at 1 mg bid and quickly increase to 2 mg bid. In elderly patients the initial dose should be 0.25–0.5 mg bid.
- Risperidone is the only atypical antipsychotic currently available in a long-acting injectable form (Risperdal Consta).
  - Patient should first be stabilized with oral medication.
  - Recommended starting dose is 25 mg regardless of the patient's previous or current oral dose of antipsychotic medication.
  - Injections are given every 2 weeks, and steady-state plasma concentrations are achieved after four injections.
  - Not much drug is released for the first 3 weeks following the injection, and oral antipsychotic supplementation is recommended.
  - Although there is an initial release of medication, the amount released is small and the main release of the drug starts from 3 weeks after the injection. This release is maintained from 4 to 6 weeks and subsides by 7 weeks.

- – If the patient has not taken risperidone before, a trial of oral risperidone is recommended to see if there is a hypersensitivity reaction.
- – Maximum dose is 50 mg every 2 weeks.

- After the first week of treatment, the entire oral dose can be given at bedtime.
- The optimal dosage in North American trials was 6 mg/day, but most patients do well at 3–6 mg/day. Elderly patients may require dosages as low as 0.5 mg/day.
- Risperidone combines dopamine D_2 receptor antagonism with potent 5-HT_2 receptor antagonism; it also antagonizes dopamine D_1 and D_4 receptors, α_1- and α_2-adrenergic receptors, and histamine H_1 receptors.
- Risperidone has the most D_2 affinity of the atypical antipsychotics.
- All three oral forms of this medication are bioequivalent.

Risks, side effects, and their management

- Insomnia, hypotension, agitation, headache, and rhinitis are the most common side effects of risperidone; they tend to decrease with time.
- Average weight gain associated with risperidone after 10 weeks of treatment is 2.10 kg.
- Unlike other atypical antipsychotics, risperidone increases prolactin levels.
- Risperidone does not have significant anticholinergic side effects.

Drug interactions

Risperidone is metabolized by CYP 2D6; medications that inhibit CYP 2D6, such as many SSRIs, cause increases in plasma levels of risperidone.

OLANZAPINE (TABLET, ORAL DISINTEGRATING TABLET, INTRAMUSCULAR ADMINISTRATION)

Clinical use

- Initial dosing: Start at 10 mg qhs for patients with schizophrenia and 15 mg qhs for acutely manic patients (single daily dose).
- The dose for maintenance treatment of bipolar disorder is 5–20 mg.

- Olanzapine is a selective monoaminergic antagonist with high affinity binding at the 5-HT$_2$ and D$_{1-4}$ receptors.
- The oral disintegrating tablet and the solution form of the medication are bioequivalent to the tablet.
- The intramuscular preparation is twice as potent as the oral forms (10 mg im is equivalent to 20 mg po).

Risks, side effects, and their management

- Somnolence and psychomotor slowing are dose dependent.
- Treatment-emergent seizures are rare in the absence of concomitant medical disorders.
- Increased transaminase levels occur in approximately 2% of patients. These levels often normalize without medication discontinuation.
- Treatment-emergent weight gain is common.
  - Weight gain averages about 4.15 kg after 10 weeks of treatment.
  - By 39 weeks, weight gain tends to plateau.
  - Approximately 20% of patients may not gain weight.
  - Weight gain is not dose dependent.

Drug interactions

- Olanzapine is metabolized by several pathways; thus, it is unlikely to be affected by concurrent administration of other medications.
- Additive pharmacodynamic effects should be expected if olanzapine is combined with medications that have anticholinergic, antihistaminic, or α_1-adrenergic side effects.

QUETIAPINE (TABLET)

Clinical use

- Initial dosing:
  - In the treatment of schizophrenia, start at 25 mg bid, with increases to 50 mg bid on day 2, 100 mg bid on day 3, and 100 mg in the morning and 200 mg in the evening on day 4.
  - In the treatment of acute mania, start with bid dosages totaling 100 mg/day on day 1, 200 mg on day 2, 300 mg on day 3, and 400 mg on day 4. Adjustments up to 800 mg/day by day 6 may be made if needed.

- Dosages should not be increased by more than 200 mg/day on days 5 and 6.

- Optimal dosage ranges from 400 mg/day to 600 mg/day.
- Quetiapine has a short half-life of 6–8 hours and is usually administered twice a day.
- Quetiapine also has FDA indication for treatment of bipolar depression.

Risks, side effects, and their management

- Somnolence is one of the most common side effects of quetiapine. Somnolence and psychomotor slowing are dose dependent. Patients usually become tolerant to these effects.
- Incidence of extrapyramidal side effects and changes in prolactin levels were the same as placebo in trials.
- Quetiapine may induce orthostatic hypotension and concomitant symptoms of dizziness, tachycardia, and syncope. The risk of symptomatic hypotension is particularly pronounced during initial dose titration.
- Increased transaminase levels have been seen in 6% of patients treated with quetiapine; the effects of these increased levels have all been benign to date.
- Use quetiapine with caution in patients with hepatic disease or risk factors for hepatic toxicity.
- A weight gain of at least 7% of base body weight was observed in 23% of patients during trials.

Drug interactions

- Quetiapine is metabolized by hepatic CYP 3A3/4.
- Concurrent administration of CYP-inducing drugs, such as carbamazepine, decreases blood levels of quetiapine.
- Quetiapine does not appreciably affect the pharmacokinetics of other medications.
- Because it may induce hypotension, quetiapine may enhance the effects of certain antihypertensive agents.

ZIPRASIDONE (CAPSULE, INTRAMUSCULAR ADMINISTRATION)

Clinical use

- Initial dosing:
  - In the treatment of schizophrenia, start at 20–40 mg bid; the dosage can be rapidly titrated to 60–80 mg bid over 2–4 days if the patient is not elderly and is healthy.
  - In the treatment of acute mania, start at 40 mg bid and increase to 60 mg or 80 mg on day 2; the dosage should be subsequently adjusted based on individual tolerance and symptoms to between 40 and 80 mg bid.

- Ziprasidone is usually given twice a day with meals; food increases absorption by approximately 100%.
- Ziprasidone is a 5-HT_{2A} and D_2 antagonist.
- The recommended dose for intramuscular injection is 10–20 mg, with a maximum dosage of 40 mg/day. It can be given 10 mg every 2 hours or 20 mg every 4 hours.

Risks, side effects, and their management

- The most common side effects of ziprasidone are headache, dyspepsia, nausea, constipation, abdominal pain, somnolence, and EPS.
- Ziprasidone produced a mean QTc prolongation of 21 milliseconds at maximal blood levels.
  - In all clinical trials, the rate of QTc intervals >500 milliseconds (considered a threshold for arrhythmia risk) did not differ from the rate associated with placebo.
  - The QTc effect of ziprasidone is larger than that of other atypical antipsychotics.

- Ziprasidone is associated with less weight gain than other atypical antipsychotics.

Drug interactions

Drugs that inhibit CYP 3A4 reduce metabolism of ziprasidone: concurrent treatment with ketoconazole increased blood levels of ziprasidone by approximately 40%. Carbamazepine (and possibly other enzyme inducers) may decrease ziprasidone blood levels by roughly 35%.

ARIPIPRAZOLE (TABLET, LIQUID)

Clinical use

- Initial dosing:
  - In the treatment of schizophrenia, start at 10 or 15 mg/day.
  - In the treatment of acute mania or mixed episodes, start at 30 mg/day.
  - In the maintenance treatment of stable patients with bipolar I disorder, start at 15 mg/day.

- Doses higher than 10–15 mg have not been shown to be more effective in patients with schizophrenia.
- Aripiprazole is FDA approved for the treatment of schizophrenia, acute mania or mixed episodes in bipolar disorder, and maintenance treatment in bipolar I disorder., and as an augmentation agent in major depression unresponsive to antidepressant treatment.
- Elimination half-life is 75 hours (longest of the atypical antipsychotics), and steady-state concentrations are reached within 2 weeks.
- At equivalent doses, plasma concentrations of the solution were higher compared with plasma concentrations associated with the tablet form.
- Aripiprazole has high affinity for dopamine D_2 and D_3 receptors and $5\text{-}HT_{1A}$ and $5\text{-}HT_{2A}$ receptors. The mechanism of action is not known, but aripiprazole may mediate its effects via a combination of partial agonist activity at the D_2 and $5\text{-}HT_{1A}$ receptors and antagonist activity at the $5\text{-}HT_{2A}$ receptors.

Risks, side effects, and their management

- The most common side effects of aripiprazole include headache, nausea, dyspepsia, agitation, anxiety, insomnia, somnolence, and akathisia.
- Akathisia may be avoided by starting at doses lower than 10 mg and increasing the dose slowly.
- Aripiprazole is not associated with significant sedation, anticholinergic side effects, weight gain, or cardiovascular side effects.

Drug interactions

- Aripiprazole is hepatically metabolized by CYP 2D6 and CYP 3A4.
- The dose should be halved when given with a CYP 3A4 inhibitor such as ketoconazole. The dose should be decreased when given with a CYP 2D6 inhibitor such as fluoxetine.
- When given with CYP 3A4 inducers such as carbamazepine, the dose of aripiprazole should be doubled.

PALIPERIDONE (TABLET, EXTENDED RELEASE)

Clinical use

- Paliperidone is the primary active metabolite of risperidone.
- Initial dosing: Start at the recommended 6-mg dose; no initial dose titration is necessary.
- Paliperidone has an extended-release formulation, and once-a-day morning dosing is recommended.
- If exceeding 6 mg/day, increases of 3 mg/day are not recommended more frequently than every 5 days, up to a maximum of 12 mg/day.
- Paliperidone has high affinity for α_1, D_2, H_1, and 5-HT_{2C} receptors.
- Compared with risperidone, paliperidone has a nearly 10-fold lower affinity for α_2 and 5-HT_{2A} receptors and a nearly three- to fivefold lower affinity for 5-HT_{1A} and 5-HT_{1D}, respectively.
- Paliperidone currently has FDA indication only for schizophrenia.

Risks, side effects, and their management

- The most common side effects of paliperidone are akathisia, EPS, tachycardia, headache, and somnolence.
- Prolactin elevation with paliperidone is similar to that seen with risperidone.

Drug interactions

- Paliperidone is hepatically metabolized by CYP 2D6 and CYP 3A4.
- The dose should be halved when given with a CYP 3A4 inhibitor such as ketoconazole. The dose should be decreased when given with a CYP 2D6 inhibitor such as fluoxetine.
- When given with CYP 3A4 inducers such as carbamazepine, the paliperidone dose should be doubled.

Conventional Antipsychotics

DRUG POTENCY

The term *drug potency* refers to the milligram equivalence of drugs, not to their relative efficacy. For example, although haloperidol is more potent than chlorpromazine (haloperidol 2 mg=chlorpromazine 100 mg), therapeutically equivalent doses are equally effective (haloperidol 12 mg=chlorpromazine 600 mg). Typically, the potency of antipsychotic drugs is compared with the potency of chlorpromazine 100 mg.

- The high-potency conventional antipsychotics are haloperidol, fluphenazine, trifluoperazine, pimozide, and thiothixene.
  - As a rule, high-potency conventional antipsychotics have an equivalent dose of less than 5 mg.
  - Compared with low-potency conventional antipsychotics, these drugs are associated with more EPS but less sedation, fewer anticholinergic side effects, and less hypotension.

- The low-potency conventional antipsychotics are chlorpromazine, mesoridazine, and thioridazine.
  - These drugs have an equivalent dose of more than 40 mg.
  - Compared with high-potency conventional antipsychotics, these drugs are associated with greater sedation, more anticholinergic side effects, and more hypotension; however, acute EPS are less frequent.

- The intermediate-potency conventional antipsychotics are loxapine, molindone, and perphenazine.
  - These drugs have an equivalent dose between 5 and 40 mg.
  - These drugs have a side-effect profile that lies between the profiles of the other two groups.

- Tardive dyskinesia rates for high- and low-potency conventional antipsychotics do not differ.
- In most circumstances in which conventional antipsychotics are used, high-potency drugs are preferred, because EPS can usually be minimized by using the lowest effective dose or by treating them symptomatically, whereas anticholinergic and autonomic side effects are potentially more dangerous and difficult to manage.

CONVENTIONAL LONG-ACTING INJECTABLE ANTIPSYCHOTICS

Many clinicians prefer to continue giving oral medication at approximately half the previous maintenance dose during the first few months of depot antipsychotic administration, rather than administer a loading dose of depot medication. Breakthrough psychotic symptoms are treated with supplemental oral medication, and the dose of the next scheduled depot injection can be increased accordingly. Side effects may take months to subside, and withdrawal dyskinesia may not appear for months after discontinuation of the decanoate formulation.

Haloperidol decanoate

- Patients receive an initial dose that is 20 times the oral maintenance dose (Ereshefsky et al. 1993).
- The maximum volume per injection of haloperidol decanoate should not exceed 3 mL, and the maximum dose per injection should not exceed 100 mg.
    - If 20 times the oral dose is greater than 100 mg, the dose is given in divided injections spaced 3–7 days apart.
- Subsequent doses are decreased monthly, to about 10 times the oral dose by the third or fourth month. Ten times the oral dose, administered every 4 weeks, is a typical maintenance dose for haloperidol decanoate.
- Steady-state serum concentrations are achieved after approximately 20 weeks.

Fluphenazine decanoate

- Most patients respond to a dose of 10–30 mg given every 2 weeks.
- Steady-state serum concentrations are achieved after approximately 10 weeks (five injection intervals).

Antidepressants

All antidepressants appear to be similarly effective for treating major depression, but individual patients may respond preferentially to one agent or another. These medications are significantly different from one another with regard to side effects, lethality in overdose, pharmacokinetics, and the ability to treat comorbid disorders. Antidepressants are also effective in the treatment of the following conditions (although the

FDA has not evaluated or approved the use of antidepressants to treat many of them):

- OCD (SSRIs and clomipramine)
- Panic disorder (tricyclic antidepressants [TCAs] and monoamine oxidase inhibitors [MAOIs])
- Generalized anxiety disorder (selective serotonin-norepinephrine reuptake inhibitors [SNRIs] and SSRIs)
- Bulimia (SSRIs)
- Dysthymia (SSRIs)
- Bipolar depression (after or with treatment with a mood stabilizer)
- Social phobia (SSRIs)
- Posttraumatic stress disorder (SSRIs)
- Irritable bowel syndrome (TCAs)
- Enuresis (TCAs)
- Neuropathic pain (TCAs, duloxetine)
- Migraine headaches (TCAs)
- Attention-deficit/hyperactivity disorder (ADHD) (bupropion)
- Autism (SSRIs)
- Late luteal phase dysphoric disorder/premenstrual dysphoric disorder (SSRIs)
- Borderline personality disorder (SSRIs)
- Smoking cessation (bupropion)
- Fibromyalgia (duloxetine)

The antidepressant classes are based on similarity of receptor effects and side effects. All are effective against depression when administered in therapeutic doses. The choice of antidepressant medication is based on the patient's psychiatric symptoms, his or her history of previous treatment response, family members' history of response, medication side-effect profiles, and comorbid disorders (see Chapter 3, Table 3–4). Augmentation strategies include lithium, liothyronine (Cytomel), stimulants, and antipsychotics.

Selective Serotonin Reuptake Inhibitors

The SSRIs include citalopram, escitalopram, fluoxetine, fluvoxamine, paroxetine, and sertraline (Table 14–3).

SIDE EFFECTS

- Mild nausea, loose bowel movements, anxiety, headache, insomnia, and increased sweating are frequent initial side effects of SSRIs. They are usually dose related and may be minimized with low initial dosing and gradual titration. These effects typically decrease after several days of treatment.
- Fluoxetine tends to be the most activating.
- Sexual dysfunction is the most common longer-term side effect (decreased libido, anorgasmia, and delayed ejaculation).
- Although rarely needed, medication that blocks the $5\text{-}HT_3$ receptor (e.g., ondansetron) can be used to reduce SSRI-induced nausea.
- Serotonin syndrome can be fatal.
  - The most common symptoms are lethargy, restlessness, confusion, flushing, diaphoresis, tremor, and myoclonic jerks. As the condition progresses, hyperthermia, hypertonicity, myoclonus, and death may occur. Chapter 12 of this volume, "Emergency Psychiatry," provides more information about serotonin syndrome.
  - Treatment involves discontinuing the serotonergic medication and administering either the $5\text{-}HT_{2A}$ antagonist cyproheptadine (12 mg, and then 2 mg every 2 hours) or second-generation antipsychotics (because of $5\text{-}HT_{2A}$ antagonist activity) (note that efficacy has not been established for these presumed antidotes).

DRUG INTERACTIONS

- SSRIs, especially fluoxetine and paroxetine, inhibit CYP, which may result in increased levels of some concomitant medications.
- SSRI and MAOI: likely from serotonin syndrome
  - If switching from an SSRI to MAOI, the SSRI must be fully eliminated. This is 5 half-lives of the SSRI: 5 weeks for fluoxetine and about 1 week for the other SSRIs.
  - If switching from an MAOI to an SSRI, a 2-week waiting period is needed to allow resynthesis of the MAO enzyme.

TABLE 14–3. Selective serotonin reuptake inhibitors

Drug	Starting Dose (MG)[a]	Usual Daily Dose (MG)	Available Oral Doses (MG)	Mean Half-Life (Hours)
Citalopram (Celexa)	20	20–40	10, 20, 40, L	35
Escitalopram (Lexapro)	10	10–20	5, 10, 20, L	32
Fluoxetine (Prozac, Sarafem)	20	20–60	10, 20, 40, L	72–144
Fluoxetine weekly (Prozac weekly)	90	90	90	72–144
Fluvoxamine controlled release (Luvox CR)	100	100–300	100, 150	16
Paroxetine (Paxil)	20	20–50	10, 20, 30, 40, L	20
Paroxetine controlled release (Paxil CR)	25	25–62.5	12.5, 25, 37.5	20
Sertraline (Zoloft)	50	50–200	25, 50, 100, L	26–66

Note. L=Liquid/oral suspension.
[a] Average starting dose.

- SSRI and triptans: Symptoms of mild to moderate serotonin syndrome have been reported, but most patients tolerate these combinations (Gardner and Lynd 1998).

Selective Serotonin-Norepinephrine Reuptake Inhibitors

Venlafaxine, desvenlafaxine, and duloxetine are selective serotonin-norepinephrine reuptake inhibitors (Table 14–4).

VENLAFAXINE

- Venlafaxine may also have a role in treating chronic pain conditions, but data are limited.
- There is a low likelihood of drug interactions with venlafaxine; it is least likely to contribute to protein-binding interactions and unlikely to inhibit CYP.
- Unlike SSRIs, venlafaxine demonstrates a positive dose-response relationship: mild depression may respond to lower doses and more severe or recurrent depression may respond better to higher doses.
- Side effects are similar to those of SSRIs: gastrointestinal symptoms, sexual dysfunction, increased sweating, and transient discontinuation symptoms.
- Dose-dependent hypertension may occur, especially at dosages higher than 300mg/day. If clinically significant treatment-emergent hypertension occurs, consider dose reduction or treatment discontinuation.

DESVENLAFAXINE

- Active metabolite of venlafaxine
- While dosing is different from venlafaxine, the range of efficacy and tolerability are similar

DULOXETINE

- Duloxetine also has FDA approval for treatment of diabetic peripheral neuropathy and fibromyalgia, independent of depression and anxiety.
- Side effects are similar to those of SSRIs; dry mouth, constipation, and increased sweating may also occur.

TABLE 14–4. Selective serotonin-norepinephrine reuptake inhibitors

Drug	Starting dose (mg)	Usual daily dose (mg)	Available oral doses (mg)	Mean half-life (hours)
Venlafaxine (Effexor)	37.5	75–225	25, 37.5, 50, 75, 100	5–11
Venlafaxine extended release (Effexor XR)	37.5	75–225	37.5, 75, 150	5–11
Desvenlafaxine extended release (Pristiq)	50	50–400	50, 100	11
Duloxetine (Cymbalta)	60	60–120	20, 30, 60	12

- Dose-dependent nausea may occur in early phases of treatment but usually subsides in 1 week.
- Duloxetine is rarely associated with increases in serum transaminase levels (typically in the first 2 months of treatment).
- Current product labeling contains a caution regarding use in patients with significant alcohol use or chronic liver disease.
- Duloxetine should not be used in patients with uncontrolled narrow-angle glaucoma.
- Duloxetine is a moderate inhibitor of CYP 2D6 and may increase levels of other medications that use this enzyme.

Bupropion

Bupropion is considered a noradrenergic-dopaminergic antidepressant (see Table 14–5).

- Relative lack of sexual side effects
- Can be added in low doses to attenuate the sexual dysfunction caused by other medications
- Is an effective aid in smoking cessation
- Facilitates dopamine transmission, thus is thought to be helpful for patients with Parkinson's disease who refuse treatment for depression

CONTRAINDICATIONS

- Seizure disorders
- Active eating disorder
- Central nervous system tumor
- History of significant head trauma

Use caution in patients who are taking other drugs that lower the seizure threshold.

SIDE EFFECTS

- Most common are initial headache, anxiety, insomnia, increased sweating, and gastrointestinal upset
- May also get tremor and akathisia

TABLE 14–5. Buproprion

Drug	Starting dose (mg)	Usual daily dose (mg)	Available oral doses (mg)	Mean half-life (hours)
Bupropion (Wellbutrin)	150	300	75, 100	14
Bupropion sustained release (Wellbutrin SR, Zyban)	150	300	100, 150	21
Bupropion extended release (Wellbutrin XL)	150	300	150, 300	21

- Reports of delusions, hallucinations, and paranoia with bupropion-mediated increases in central dopamine; use with caution in patients with psychotic disorders

Serotonin Modulators

Nefazodone and trazodone are serotonin modulators (Table 14–6).

NEFAZODONE

- Nefazodone is primarily a postsynaptic 5-HT$_2$ antagonist.
- The generic formulation is available, but the branded product was removed from the market in 2003 after reports of hepatotoxicity.
- This medication is mostly for patients who are currently stable on the medication and want to continue this treatment rather than switch to an alternative agent.
- If there is an increase in serum transaminase levels that is three times the upper limits of the normal range or higher, patient should be withdrawn from nefazodone and should not be considered for rechallenge.
- Coadministration with most medications that are metabolized by CYP 3A3/4 should be undertaken with caution.

TRAZODONE

- Trazodone is associated with significant sedation, which has led some clinicians to combine low dosages (50–100 mg) with other nonsedating antidepressant medications for nonspecific insomnia. However, little data is available to support the use of this agent as a hypnotic.
- Trazodone is not recommended as a first-line antidepressant.
- Adverse effects include orthostatic hypotension, arrhythmias, and priapism. Priapism may be irreversible and require surgery; be sure to inform patients of this risk.
- Myocardial irritation may occur in overdose if the patient has preexisting ventricular conduction abnormalities.

Norepinephrine-Serotonin Modulators

Mirtazapine (Remeron) is a norepinephrine-serotonin modulator (Table 14–7).

TABLE 14–6. Serotonin modulators

Drug	Starting dose (mg)	Usual daily dose (mg)	Available oral doses (mg)	Mean half-life (hours)
Nefazodone (Serzone)	50	150–300	100, 150, 200, 250	4
Trazodone (Desyrel)	50	75–300	50, 100, 150, 300	7

Note. Only generic available in U.S.

TABLE 14–7. Norepinephrine-serotonin modulators

Drug	Starting dose (mg)	Usual daily dose (mg)	Available oral doses (mg)	Mean half-life (hours)
Mirtazapine (Remeron)	15	15–45	15, 30, 45	20

- Mirtazapine reduces anxiety and sleep disturbances in depressed patients as early as 1 week after beginning the medication.

- Adverse effects include weight gain, sedation, hypertension, vasodilation with peripheral edema, dizziness, dry mouth, and constipation (anticholinergic). There is minimal sexual dysfunction and minimal nausea.

- Mirtazapine is unlikely to be associated with CYP-mediated drug interaction.

- Clinical trials showed that 3 of 2,796 patients developed agranulocytosis/neutropenia. Routine monitoring is not recommended.

- Do not use with an MAOI or within 14 days of discontinuing an MAOI.

Tricyclic and Heterocyclic Antidepressants

The tricyclic and heterocyclic antidepressants include amitriptyline, clomipramine, doxepin, imipramine, trimipramine, desipramine, nortriptyline, protriptyline, amoxapine, and maprotiline (Table 14–8).

- TCAs may be more effective than SSRIs in the treatment of major depression with melancholic features.

- A baseline electrocardiogram should be ordered if the patient has heart disease or is over 40 years old.

- Tertiary amine TCAs have more potent serotonin reuptake inhibition and tend to have more side effects than secondary amine TCAs.

- Secondary amine TCAs have more potent noradrenergic reuptake inhibition than tertiary amine TCAs.

- Clinically meaningful plasma levels are available for imipramine, desipramine, and nortriptyline only. Blood should be drawn approximately 10–14 hours after the last dose of medication.

- Patients with significant anxiety, panic, or a tendency to be sensitive to side effects should receive a 50% lower initial dose. Also, lower initial doses are recommended in elderly patients and those with cardiovascular or hepatic disease.

- Desipramine and protriptyline tend to be activating. Trimipramine, amitriptyline, and doxepin are the most sedating.

TABLE 14–8. Tricyclic and heterocyclic antidepressants

Drug	Starting dose (mg)	Usual daily dose (mg)	Available oral doses (mg)	Mean half-life (hours)
Tricyclics				
Tertiary amine tricyclics				
Amitriptyline (Elavil)	25–50	100–300	10, 25, 50, 75, 100, 150	15.6–26.6
Clomipramine (Anafranil)	25	100–250	25, 50, 75	32–69
Doxepin (Sinequan)	25–50	100–300	10, 25, 50, 75, 100, 150	16.8
Imipramine (Tofranil, Tofranil-PM)	25–50	100–300	10, 25, 50, 75, 100, 125, 150	7.6–17.1
Trimipramine (Surmontil)	25–50	100–300	25, 50, 100	24
Secondary amine tricyclics				
Desipramine (Norpramin)	25–50	100–300	25, 50, 75, 100, 150	17.1
Nortriptyline (Pamelor)	25	50–150	10, 25, 50, 75	26.6
Protriptyline (Vivactil)	10	15–60	5, 10	78.4
Tetracyclics				
Amoxapine (Asendin)	50	100–400	25, 50, 100, 150	8
Maprotiline (generic)	50	100–225	25, 50, 75	43

SIDE EFFECTS

- Amoxapine antagonizes D_2 receptors and can cause EPS, aka-thisia, and even tardive dyskinesia.
- Among drugs in this class, nortriptyline is the least likely to produce orthostatic hypotension.

Anticholinergic effects

- Use these drugs with caution in patients with prostatic hypertrophy, narrow-angle glaucoma, or cognitive impairment.
- The most common anticholinergic side effects are dry mouth, constipation, urinary retention, blurred vision, and tachycardia.
- Drugs in this class may cause cognitive impairment and confusion in the elderly.
- Anticholinergic effects result from antagonism of muscarinic receptors.
- Tertiary amines and protriptyline have a particularly high affinity for muscarinic receptors and are more likely than other tricyclic antidepressants to have anticholinergic side effects.
- Pilocarpine oral rinse or eyedrops can be helpful for local relief of symptoms.
- Consider cholinergic medication (bethanechol 10–15 mg po tid–qid) only after dose reduction and trying an alternative antidepressant with fewer anticholinergic side effects.

Cardiovascular effects

- This class of drugs can cause orthostatic hypotension, tachycardia, and cardiac conduction delays; in overdose they can cause life-threatening arrhythmias.
- PR and QRS intervals are prolonged.
- Avoid these drugs in patients with bundle branch block, because use can lead to life-threatening second- or third-degree heart block.

Weight gain

- Weight gain is common with this class of drugs. Secondary amines are less likely than tertiary amines to produce weight gain.

Seizures

- Dose-related risk of seizures has been found with clomipramine; the daily dose should not exceed 250 mg.
- Overdoses, particularly of amoxapine and desipramine, are associated with seizures.
- It is controversial whether therapeutic doses lower the seizure threshold; other classes of medications are safer for patients with epilepsy.
- When the QRS interval is less than 0.10 second, the likelihood of ventricular arrhythmias decreases.

OVERDOSE

- Tricyclic antidepressants have anticholinergic activity, which leads to agitation, supraventricular arrhythmias, hallucinations, severe hypertension, seizures, and anticholinergic delirium in overdose.
- Patients with anticholinergic delirium have hot, dry skin; dry mucous membranes; dilated pupils; absent bowel sounds; confusion; and tachycardia. Anticholinergic delirium is a medical emergency.
- Hypotension, which may result from norepinephrine depletion, should be treated with vigorous intravenous fluid.

DRUG INTERACTIONS

- TCAs are metabolized by the liver; CYP 2D6 inhibitors may significantly increase TCA levels.
- TCAs rarely affect the metabolism of other drugs; however, valproate sodium may have decreased levels when given with TCAs.
- Guanethidine and clonidine lose effectiveness if administered concomitantly with TCAs.

DOSING GUIDELINES

Nortriptyline

- This drug should be initiated at 25 mg/day and increased to 75 mg/day over 1–2 weeks.
- The therapeutic plasma level is between 50 and 150 ng/mL.

Amitriptyline, clomipramine, doxepin, imipramine, trimipramine, and desipramine

- Can be initiated at 25–50 mg/day. Divided dosing may be used at first to minimize side effects, but eventually the entire dose can be given at bedtime. The dosage can be increased to 150 mg/day the second week, 225 mg/day the third week, and 300 mg/day the fourth week.
- Clomipramine should not exceed 250 mg/day because of an increased risk of seizures at a higher dose.
- Therapeutic plasma levels (reached after 5–7 days):
  - For imipramine, the sum of the plasma levels of imipramine and the desmethyl metabolite (desipramine) should be greater than 200–250 ng/mL.
  - For desipramine, levels should be greater than 125 ng/mL.

Protriptyline

- This drug can be initiated at 10 mg/day; the maximum dosage is 60 mg/day.
- This drug tends to be activating.

Amoxapine

- This drug has an active metabolite that antagonizes dopamine D_2 receptors and can cause treatment-emergent EPS.
- This drug has a short half-life and should be given in divided doses.

Maprotiline

- This drug can be initiated at 50 mg/day, and that dosage should be maintained for 2 weeks.
- There is increased risk of seizure if the dosage is raised too quickly.
- The dosage can be increased over 4 weeks to 225 mg/day.

Monoamine Oxidase Inhibitors

The MAOIs include phenelzine, tranylcypromine, and selegiline; the last three are irreversible nonselective MAOIs (Table 14–9).

- The MAOIs are not currently used as first-line agents.

TABLE 14–9. Irreversible, nonselective monoamine oxidase inhibitors

DRUG	STARTING DOSE (MG)	USUAL DAILY DOSE (MG)	AVAILABLE DOSES (MG)	MEAN HALF-LIFE (HOURS)
Phenelzine (Nardil)	15	15–90	15	2
Tranylcypromine (Parnate)	10	30–60	10	2
Selegiline transdermal system (Emsam)	6/24-hour patch		6-, 9-, 12/24-hour patch	18–25

- Patients with atypical depression show a preferential response to MAOI therapy (Liebowitz et al. 1984; Quitkin et al. 1979; Ravaris et al. 1980; Zisook 1985).
- Patients should be educated to notify their physicians that they are taking MAOIs before accepting any medication or anesthetic.
- Monoamine oxidase A (MAO A) inhibition appears to be most relevant to the antidepressant effects of these drugs.
- Drugs that inhibit both MAO A and monoamine oxidase B (MAO B) are called nonselective. The MAOI antidepressants currently available in the United States are nonselective inhibitors.
- Because the enzyme needs to be resynthesized, a period of 10–14 days is required after discontinuing irreversible inhibitors and before instituting treatment with other antidepressants or permitting the use of contraindicated drugs or the consumption of contraindicated foods.
- The importance of complying with dietary and medication restrictions (Table 14–10) should be discussed with the patient when nonselective MAOIs are being used; Table 14–11 lists the necessary instructions.
- After tolerance to the hypotensive side effects has developed (usually after 1 or 2 weeks), the medication can be taken in a single daily dose in the morning. Morning dosing is preferred because MAOIs tend to be activating.

SIDE EFFECTS

- The most common side effects seen with this class of drugs are orthostatic hypotension, headache, insomnia, weight gain, sexual dysfunction, peripheral edema, and afternoon somnolence.
- Anticholinergic-like side effects are present at the beginning of treatment, even though there is no significant affinity for muscarinic receptors.

Hypertensive crisis

- Large amounts of dietary tyramine can result in a hypertensive crisis in patients taking MAOIs, because increased amounts of norepinephrine result in profound α-adrenergic activation.

TABLE 14–10.   Dietary and medication restrictions for patients taking nonselective monoamine oxidase inhibitors (MAOIs)

FOODS		DRUGS	
AVOID[a]	SAFE	AVOID[a]	SAFE
Aged cheeses	Alcohol (but not tap beer), in moderation	All sympathomimetic and stimulant drugs, including	Cold and allergy medications
Aged or fermented meats (e.g., sausage, salami, pepperoni)	Fresh cheeses (e.g., cream cheese, cottage cheese, ricotta cheese, American cheese, moderate	Amphetamines	Alka-Seltzer (plain)
All foods that may be spoiled	amounts of mozzarella)	Buspirone	Chlor-Trimeton Allergy (without decongestant)
Fava beans and broad bean pods	Fresh yogurt	Diet medications	Robitussin (plain)
Meat extracts (i.e., Bovril)	Smoked salmon and whitefish	Ephedrine	Steroid inhalers
Sauerkraut	Yeast and baked goods containing yeast	Fenfluramine and dexfenfluramine	Tylenol (plain)
Soy sauce		Isoproterenol	Other
Tap beer, including nonalcoholic tap beer		L-dopa and dopamine	Antibiotics
Yeast extracts (i.e., Marmite)		Local anesthetic drugs containing ephedrine or cocaine	Codeine
		Meperidine	Laxatives and stool softeners
		Methylphenidate	Local anesthetics without epinephrine or cocaine
		Other antidepressant medications	Morphine
		Phenylephrine	Nonsteroidal anti-inflammatory drugs
		Phenylpropanolamine	

TABLE 14–10. Dietary and medication restrictions for patients taking nonselective monoamine oxidase inhibitors (MAOIs) *(continued)*

FOODS		DRUGS	
AVOID[a]	SAFE	AVOID[a]	SAFE
		Over-the-counter nasal decongestants and cold, sinus, and allergy medications containing pseudoephedrine, phenylephrine, or phenylpropanolamine	Robitussin CF, DM, Night Relief, PE
		Actifed	Sine-Aid
		Alka-Seltzer Plus	Sine-Off
		Allerest	Sinex
		Contac	Triaminic
		Coricidin D	Tylenol
		CoTylenol	Vicks 44D, 44M
		Dristan	
		Neo-Synephrine	
		NyQuil	

[a]Avoid while taking a monoamine oxidase inhibitor and for 2 weeks after discontinuing the medication.

TABLE 14–11. **Instructions for patients taking nonselective monoamine oxidase inhibitors**

- Avoid all foods and drugs on the list (see Table 14–10).

- In general, all foods you should avoid are decayed, fermented, or aged in some way. Avoid any spoiled food, even if it is not on the list.

- If you get a cold or the flu, you may take aspirin or Tylenol. For a cough, glycerin cough drops or cough syrup without dextromethorphan may be used.

- All laxatives and stool softeners may be used.

- For infections, all antibiotics (such as penicillin, tetracycline, or erythromycin) may be safely prescribed.

- Do not take any other medications without first checking with your doctor. These medications include over-the-counter medicines bought without prescription, such as cold tablets, nose drops, cough medicine, and diet pills.

- Eating one of the restricted foods may suddenly increase your blood pressure. If this occurs, you will get an explosive headache, particularly in the back of your head and in your temples. Your head and face will feel flushed and full, your heart may pound, and you may perspire heavily and feel nauseated. If this rare reaction occurs, do not lie down, because this increases your blood pressure further. If your blood pressure is high, go to the nearest emergency center for evaluation and treatment. Do not wait for a returned phone call from the doctor's office.

- If you need dental care or medical care from another doctor while taking this medication, show these restrictions and instructions to the dentist or doctor. Have the dentist or doctor call your regular doctor's office if he or she has any questions or needs further clarification or information.

- Side effects such as postural light-headedness, constipation, delay in urination, delay in ejaculation and orgasm, muscle twitching, sedation, fluid retention, insomnia, and excessive sweating are quite common. Many of these side effects lessen after the third week.

- Light-headedness may occur after sudden changes in position. It can be avoided by getting up slowly. If tablets are taken with meals, this and the other side effects are lessened.

TABLE 14–11. Instructions for patients taking nonselective monoamine oxidase inhibitors *(continued)*

- The medication is rarely effective in less than 3 weeks.

- Care should be taken while operating any machinery or driving; some patients have episodes of sleepiness in the early phase of treatment.

- Take the medication precisely as directed. Do not regulate the number of pills without first consulting your doctor.

- In spite of the side effects and special dietary restrictions, your medication (a monoamine oxidase inhibitor) is safe and effective when taken as directed.

- If any special problems arise, call your doctor.

Source. Adapted from Jenike 1987.

- The key foods to avoid are aged cheeses, fermented sausage, sauerkraut, soy sauce, yeast extracts such as Marmite, fava beans (also called broad beans), and any foods that are overripe or spoiled.

- Fresh, unaged cheeses—such as cottage cheese, ricotta, and cream cheese—are safe.

- There are reports of spontaneous hypertension associated with MAOI therapy even when the patient is compliant with restrictions.

- A mild reaction may consist of sweating, palpitations, and a slight headache.

- A hypertensive crisis consists of severe headache, increased blood pressure, and possible intracerebral hemorrhage.

- When a patient who is being treated with an MAOI develops a headache, he or she should check blood pressure at home to determine whether a true hypertensive crisis might be occurring.

- Treatments for MAOI-induced hypertension include administration of the calcium channel blocker nifedipine and use of drugs with α-adrenergic–blocking properties, such as phentolamine (Regitine, 5 mg iv). Treatment should take place in an emergency room setting because treatment is associated with cardiac arrhythmias or severe hypotension.

Serotonin syndrome

- See the section on SSRIs earlier in this chapter for a description of the serotonin syndrome, treatment guidelines, and guidelines for switching from SSRIs to MAOIs and vice versa.
- The combination of MAOIs with meperidine (Demerol), and perhaps with other phenylpiperidine analgesics, has also been implicated in fatal reactions attributed to the serotonin syndrome.
- Of the narcotic agents, codeine and morphine are safe in combination with MAOIs, but lower doses may need to be used.

Cardiovascular effects

- MAOIs cause significant hypotension, which is often the dose-limiting side effect of these drugs.
- Expansion of intravascular volume with the use of salt tablets or fludrocortisone may be effective.

Central nervous system effects

- Headache and insomnia are common initial side effects that usually disappear after the first few weeks of treatment.

Weight gain

- Significant weight gain is a common side effect of MAOIs.

Sexual dysfunction

- Sexual side effects seen with MAOIs include decreased libido, delayed ejaculation, anorgasmia, and impotence.

DOSING GUIDELINES

Phenelzine

- Initiate at a dose of 15 mg in the morning; increase by 15 mg every other day until a total daily dose of 60 mg is reached.
- If no response occurs within 2 weeks, the dosage may be increased in 15-mg increments to a usual maximum of 90 mg/day.
- Higher doses are sometimes used, if tolerated, in patients with severe, refractory depression.

Tranylcypromine

- Initiate at a dose of 10 mg; increase every other day until 30 mg/day is reached.
- Higher doses may be necessary when the condition is refractory to treatment.

Selegiline transdermal system

- No dietary restrictions with the 6-mg/24-hour dosage; dietary modifications are required with 9-mg/24-hour and 12-mg/24-hour dosages.

Mood Stabilizers

Lithium

INDICATIONS

- Lithium is effective for acute and prophylactic treatment of manic and depressive episodes in bipolar disorder.
- Patients with rapid-cycling bipolar disorder (four or more mood disorder episodes per year) respond less well to lithium.
- Lithium is more effective at treating manic symptoms than at treating depressive symptoms of bipolar disorder.
- Lithium is effective in depressive-episode prophylaxis in patients with recurrent unipolar depression.
- Lithium may help maintain remission of depressive episodes after electroconvulsive therapy.
- Lithium may also be used in the treatment of aggression and behavioral dyscontrol.

CLINICAL USE

- The half-life of lithium is 24 hours.
- Lithium can be administered as a single daily dose because of its half-life. Evening dosing is preferred because side effects are more prevalent during peak blood levels.
- Steady-state concentrations are reached in about 5 days, which is when plasma levels should be checked. Labs should be drawn 12 hours after the last dose.

- Therapeutic plasma levels are 0.5–1.2 mEq/L. Levels of at least 0.8 mEq/L are often required in the treatment of acute manic episodes. For prophylaxis, levels of 0.6–0.8 mEq/L are commonly used to balance risks and benefits.

- Once the therapeutic level is reached, check plasma level every month for 3 months and then every 3 months thereafter.

- Initial evaluation (labs) should include thyroid function, renal panel, pregnancy test in females, and electrocardiogram in any patient with cardiac risk factors or over the age of 40 years.

- Check blood urea nitrogen (BUN) and creatinine prior to initiation of lithium and every 3–6 months.

CONTRAINDICATIONS

- Lithium should not be used in those with unstable renal function or in those with sinus node dysfunction (sick sinus syndrome).

- The risk of Ebstein anomaly for infants exposed in utero is 0.1%–0.7% (vs. a 0.1% risk of this anomaly in the general population).

RISKS AND SIDE EFFECTS

- Renal: Lithium inhibits vasopressin, which impairs the kidney's concentrating ability (nephrogenic diabetes insipidus) and results in polyuria in up to 60% of patients; this condition may be treated with diuretics.
  - Thiazides may increase lithium levels to the toxic range.
  - Amiloride 5 mg bid blocks absorption of lithium in the renal tubules.

- Thyroid dysfunction
  - Lithium causes reversible hypothyroidism in as many as 20% of patients; this is more likely in females.
  - Thyroid function should be evaluated every 6–12 months or if symptoms that might be due to thyroid dysfunction develop, including depression and rapid cycling.

- Parathyroid dysfunction
  - Patients taking lithium can have hyperparathyroidism that results in hypercalcemia and causes back pain, kyphoscoliosis,

osteoporosis, hypertension, cardiomegaly, and impaired renal function.

- If patient is symptomatic, check serum calcium ion levels.

- Neurotoxicity
  - A fine resting tremor is common. Use beta-blockers such as propranolol (<80 mg/day in divided doses).
  - Subjective memory impairment is a frequent reason for non-compliance.

- Cardiac effects
  - Benign flattening of T waves is seen in 20%–30% of patients taking lithium.
  - Lithium may suppress sinus node and cause sinoatrial block.
  - If the patient is older than 40 years or has cardiac disease, obtain a baseline electrocardiogram.

- Weight gain
- Dermatological: Acne, follicular eruptions, psoriasis, hair loss, and thinning are associated with lithium.
- Gastrointestinal
  - Nausea and diarrhea may be experienced early in treatment.
  - Side effects may improve if medication is taken with meals
  - Immediate-release preparations are more associated with nausea, and sustained-release preparations are more associated with diarrhea.

- Hematological: Leukocytosis (15,000 WBC/mm^3) is usually benign and reversible.

TOXICITY

Emphasize prevention of toxicity by encouraging adequate salt and water intake, especially during exercise and hot weather. Toxic lithium levels can cause dysarthria, ataxia, and intention tremor (see Chapter 12, "Emergency Psychiatry").

DRUG INTERACTIONS

- Thiazides reduce lithium clearance and may increase levels; this does not occur with loop diuretics.
- Nonsteroidal anti-inflammatory drugs may increase levels by decreasing lithium clearance.
- Angiotensin-converting enzyme (ACE) inhibitors and cyclooxygenase-2 (COX-2) inhibitors may increase lithium serum levels.
- Theophylline and aminophylline decrease lithium levels.
- Lithium may potentiate the effects of succinylcholine-like muscle relaxants.

Valproate

Valproate preparations include valproic acid, sodium valproate, divalproex sodium, and extended-release divalproex sodium.

INDICATIONS

- Commonly used for all phases of bipolar disorder
- Also used for mood instability from other causes

CLINICAL USE

- The half-life is 9–16 hours.
- The dosage can be initiated gradually, or a rapid loading strategy can be used.
- The dosage is usually started at 250 mg tid, with an increase of 250 mg every 3 days.
- Most patients require a daily dose of 1,250–2,000 mg.
- Moderate doses may be given once a day at bedtime to minimize daytime sedation.
- If rapid stabilization is needed, 25 mg/kg can be given.
- Plasma levels of 85–125 µg/mL are recommended for acute mania.
- The extended-release formulation has 80%–90% of the bioavailability and may require higher dosaging.
- Initial evaluation should include liver function tests, complete blood count (CBC), and pregnancy test in females.

CONTRAINDICATIONS

- Contraindicated in patients with hepatitis or liver disease
- Linked to spina bifida and other neural tube defects when infants are exposed during the first trimester

RISKS AND SIDE EFFECTS

- Hepatic toxicity
  - It is estimated that 1 in 118,000 patients taking valproate die from non-dose-related hepatic failure. No cases have been seen in patients older than 10 years, but baseline liver function tests are indicated in all patients regardless of age.
  - It is not necessary to discontinue valproate unless the increase in liver enzymes is greater than three times the upper limit of normal.
  - Increases in transaminase levels are often dose dependent.
  - Plasma ammonia levels may be transiently increased, but this increase does not require discontinuation.
  - γ-Glutamyl transferase (GGT) is often elevated with valproate therapy and is usually not clinically significant.

- Hematological
  - Hematological side effects are associated with changes in platelet counts, but thrombocytopenia is rare.
  - Coagulation defects have been reported but are rare.
  - If anticoagulation is strictly contraindicated or if the patient is on anticoagulation therapy, the coagulation profile should be checked at baseline, after 1 month, and then every 3 months.

- Gastrointestinal
  - Indigestion, heartburn, and nausea are common side effects.
  - The divalproex sodium preparation and dosing with food mitigate the gastrointestinal side effects.
  - Pancreatitis is a rare side effect when high doses are used.

- Weight gain: significant weight gain with associated hyperinsulinemia that is not dose dependent

- Neurological effects
  - Benign essential tremor
  - Drowsiness is common but subsides once steady state is reached. Once-daily dosing at bedtime may also help with daytime drowsiness.

- Alopecia: may benefit from zinc supplementation, 22.5 mg/day
- Polycystic ovarian syndrome

OVERDOSE

- Overdose results in sedation, confusion, and, ultimately, coma.
- Patient may also have hyper/hyporeflexia, seizures, respiratory suppression, and supraventricular tachycardia.

DRUG INTERACTIONS

- Valproate inhibits hepatic enzymes.
- Valproate is highly bound to plasma proteins and may displace other highly protein-bound drugs.
- Drugs that increase valproate levels are cimetidine, macrolide antibiotics (erythromycin), and felbamate.
- Valproate may increase concentrations of phenobarbital, ethosuximide, and the active 10,11-epoxide metabolite of carbamazepine, thus increasing the risk of toxicity. It may also raise the levels of lamotrigine.
- Valproate metabolism may be induced by other anticonvulsants such as carbamazepine, phenytoin, primidone, and phenobarbital, thus increasing clearance of valproate and reducing efficacy.

Carbamazepine

Tegretol and Equetro (extended release) are trade names for carbamazepine.

INDICATIONS

Carbamazepine is effective in both acute and prophylactic treatment of mania.

CLINICAL USE

- Initiate at 200 mg twice a day, and increase in 200 mg/day increments every 3–5 days; titration should be slower if the patient experiences many side effects.
- Therapeutic plasma levels are 8–12 µg/mL (based on patients treated for seizures); titrate to desired clinical response with minimal side effects.
- Patients may be prone to side effects of sedation, dizziness, and ataxia during titration phase.
- Carbamazepine induces its own metabolism (autoinduction), so dose titration may be required for weeks or months to maintain therapeutic levels; blood levels will typically decrease after 2–4 weeks of treatment.
- Initial evaluation (labs) should include alanine transaminase (ALT), aspartate transaminase (AST), CBC, pregnancy test, and sodium level.

CONTRAINDICATIONS

- Because of hematological and hepatic toxicity, avoid carbamazepine in patients with liver disease or thrombocytopenia, and those at risk for agranulocytosis; carbamazepine is strictly contraindicated in patients receiving clozapine.
- Carbamazepine is contraindicated in pregnant patients because of increased risk of spina bifida, microcephaly, and craniofacial defects with in utero exposure.

RISKS AND SIDE EFFECTS

- Hematological
  - Carbamazepine can rarely cause agranulocytosis and aplastic anemia.
  - Leukopenia, thrombocytopenia, and mild anemia occur more frequently.
  - There is no benefit to ongoing monitoring of hematological functioning if there is no clinical indication.
  - The onset of carbamazepine-induced agranulocytosis is rapid; thus, patients should be educated about the signs and symptoms of thrombocytopenia and agranulocytosis.

- Hepatic
  - Carbamazepine is occasionally associated with a hypersensitivity hepatitis that appears after a latency period of several weeks and involves increases in ALT, AST, and lactate dehydrogenase (LDH).
  - Cholestasis is also possible, with increases in bilirubin and alkaline phosphatase.
  - Mild, transient increases in transaminase levels generally do not necessitate discontinuation of carbamazepine. If ALT or AST levels increase more than three times the upper limit of normal, carbamazepine should be discontinued.

- Dermatological
  - Rash is a common side effect, occurring in 3%–17% of patients taking carbamazepine; and typically occurs within 2–20 weeks after treatment initiation. The medication is usually discontinued if a rash develops, because of the risk of progression to exfoliative dermatitis or Stevens-Johnson syndrome.

- Thyroid
  - May cause reduction in circulating thyroid hormones
  - May induce SIADH (syndrome of inappropriate antidiuretic hormone) with resultant hyponatremia

- Gastrointestinal: Nausea and occasional vomiting may be common.
- Neurological: Patients may develop dizziness, drowsiness, or ataxia, particularly during the early phases of treatment; reduce the dose and use a slower titration schedule if this occurs.

OVERDOSE

- Patients with carbamazepine overdose initially present with neuromuscular disturbances, such as nystagmus, myoclonus, and hyperreflexia, which may then progress to seizures and coma.
- Cardiac conduction changes, nausea, vomiting, and urinary retention also may occur.
- Treatment of overdose should include induction of vomiting, gastric lavage, and supportive care.

- Blood pressure, cardiac, respiratory, and kidney function should be monitored for several days after a serious overdose.

Drug Interactions

- Carbamazepine induces hepatic CYP enzymes. Medications or substances that inhibit CYP 3A3/4 may result in significant increases in plasma carbamazepine levels.
- Oral contraceptive failure may occur in patients taking carbamazepine.

Lamotrigine

Indications

- Lamotrigine is approved for the prevention of mania and depression in bipolar disorder.
- Lamotrigine is not effective in the acute treatment of mania.
- In clinical trials, it was predominantly effective in the prevention of depression.

Clinical Use

- Lamotrigine requires slow dose titration to minimize the risk of skin rash: Initiate at 25 mg/day, then increase to 50 mg/day after 2 weeks for another 2 weeks; at week 5, the dosage can be increased to 100 mg/day, and at week 6 to 200 mg/day. It is essential to follow this titration schedule regardless of the severity of illness.
- For patients taking valproate or any medication that decreases the clearance of lamotrigine, the dosing schedule and target dose should be halved.
- The titration schedule and target dose should be increased twofold in patients taking carbamazepine.
- Lamotrigine is mildly activating in many patients and thus should be dosed in the morning.

Risks and Side Effects

Lamotrigine is well tolerated and not associated with hepatotoxicity, weight gain, or significant sedation. Common early side effects include headache, dizziness, gastrointestinal distress, and blurred or double vision. The most serious side effect is rash.

- A maculopapular rash develops in 5%–10% of patients taking lamotrigine, usually in the first 8 weeks of treatment.
- Lamotrigine has also been associated with serious rashes requiring hospitalization and discontinuation of treatment. The incidence of these rashes, which have included Stevens-Johnson syndrome, is approximately 0.3% in adults on adjunctive treatment for epilepsy, 0.13% in mood disorders clinical trials of adults receiving adjunctive therapy, and 0.08% in mood disorders clinical trials in adults receiving lamotrigine as initial monotherapy (Lamictal 2005).
- Prior to initiating lamotrigine, the patient should be educated about the potential risk of developing a serious rash and the necessity to call the clinician immediately if a rash emerges.
- Development of a rash with concomitant systemic symptoms is a particularly ominous sign, and the patient should be evaluated immediately.
- Ketter et al. (2005) reported a decreased incidence of treatment-emergent rash when patients starting lamotrigine were advised to avoid other new medicines and new foods, cosmetics, conditioners, deodorants, detergents, and fabric softeners, as well as sunburn and exposure to poison ivy and poison oak. Ketter and colleagues further recommended not starting lamotrigine within 2 weeks of a rash, viral syndrome, or vaccination.

TERATOGENICITY

The North American AED Pregnancy Registry reported five cases of oral clefts in infants from a total of 684 in utero exposures to lamotrigine monotherapy (7.3/1,000) (Holmes et al. 2008).

DRUG INTERACTIONS

- Oral contraceptives can decrease concentrations of lamotrigine.
    - Lamotrigine should be carefully increased to compensate for this interaction.
    - Conversely, if the oral contraceptive is discontinued, the dose of lamotrigine should be decreased.
    - Lamotrigine does not affect the availability of oral contraceptives.

- Valproate increases lamotrigine levels.
- Carbamazepine decreases lamotrigine levels.

Oxcarbazepine

Oxcarbazepine is a keto derivative of carbamazepine, but it does not require CBC, hepatic monitoring, or serum level monitoring.

- Oxcarbazepine does not induce its own metabolism.
- It may decrease the effectiveness of oral contraceptives.
- The medication is typically initiated at 150 mg bid and titrated by 300 mg/day at weekly intervals. Therapeutic dosages are in the range of 450–1,200 mg bid.
- The conversion from carbamazepine to oxcarbazepine is at a daily dose ratio of approximately 1:1.5.
- Side effects of oxcarbazepine include hyponatremia and Stevens-Johnson syndrome.

Anxiolytics, Sedatives, and Hypnotics

Anxiety and insomnia are prevalent symptoms with multiple etiologies. Effective treatments are available, but they vary by diagnosis. In most instances, the best course of action is to treat the underlying disorder, rather than reflexively institute treatment with a nonspecific anxiolytic. Many antidepressant medications are also effective in the treatment of anxiety disorders (see Chapter 4, Table 4–4). Table 14–12 lists some commonly used anxiolytic and hypnotic medications.

Benzodiazepines

Benzodiazepines facilitate inhibition by γ-aminobutyric acid (GABA), the major inhibitory neurotransmitter in the brain. The benzodiazepine receptor is a subtype of the $GABA_A$ receptor. Benzodiazepines act rapidly because ion channels can open and close relatively quickly.

INDICATIONS

- Benzodiazepines are highly effective anxiolytics and sedatives. They also have muscle relaxant, amnestic, and anticonvulsant properties.

TABLE 14–12. Commonly used anxiolytic and hypnotic medications

DRUG	SINGLE DOSE (MG)	USUAL THERAPEUTIC DOSAGE (MG/DAY)	APPROXIMATE DOSE EQUIVALENT (MG)	METHODS OF ADMINISTRATION AND SUPPLIED FORMS	APPROXIMATE ELIMINATION HALF-LIFE, INCLUDING METABOLITES[a]
Benzodiazepines					
Alprazolam (Xanax)	0.25–1	14	0.5	po: 0.25, 0.5 mg	12 hours
Chlordiazepoxide (Librium)	5–25	15–100	10	po: 5, 10, 25 mg; iv, im[b]	14 days
Conazepam (Klonopin)	0.5–2	14	0.25	po: 0.5, 2 mg	12 days
Clorazepate (Tranxene)	3.75–22.5	15–60	7.5	po: 3.75, 7.5, 30 mg	24 days
Diazepam (Valium)	2–10	4–40	5	po: 2, 5, 10 mg; iv, im[b]	24 days
Lorazepam (Ativan)	0.5–2	1–6	1	po, sl: 0.5, 1, 2 mg; iv, im[b]	12 hours
Oxazepam (Serax)	10–30	30–120	15	po: 10,15, 30 mg	12 hours
Nonbenzodiazepines					
Buspirone (BuSpar)	10–30	30–60	N/A	po: 5, 10, 15 mg	23 hours

Note. im=intramuscular; iv=intravenous; N/A=not applicable; po=orally; sl=sublingual.
[a]The clinical duration of action of benzodiazepines does not correlate with the elimination half-life.
[b]Intramuscular lorazepam is well absorbed. Intramuscular chlordiazepoxide or diazepam is not recommended.
Source. Adapted from Teboul and Chouinard 1990.

- These medications effectively treat both acute and chronic generalized anxiety and panic disorder.
- Although only a few benzodiazepines are specifically approved by the FDA for the treatment of insomnia, almost all may be used for this purpose.
- Benzodiazepines are most clearly valuable as hypnotics in the hospital setting, where high levels of sensory stimulation, pain, and acute stress may interfere with sleep.
- Benzodiazepines are used to treat akathisia and catatonia.
- Benzodiazepines are used as adjuncts in the treatment of acute mania.
- Because alcohol and barbiturates also act, in part, via the $GABA_A$ receptor–mediated chloride ion channel, benzodiazepines exhibit cross-tolerance with these substances. Thus, benzodiazepines are used frequently for treating alcohol or barbiturate withdrawal and detoxification. Note that alcohol and barbiturates are more dangerous than benzodiazepines because they can act directly at the chloride ion channel at higher doses. In contrast, benzodiazepines have no direct effect on the ion channel; the effects of benzodiazepines are limited by the amount of endogenous GABA.

SELECTION

- At equipotent doses, all benzodiazepines have similar effects.
- The choice of benzodiazepine is generally based on half-life, rapidity of onset, metabolism, and potency.

RISKS, SIDE EFFECTS, AND THEIR MANAGEMENT

- All benzodiazepines will be metabolized at various levels by the liver, which leads to an increased risk of sedation and confusion in hepatic failure.
- Lorazepam and oxazepam are predominantly eliminated by renal excretion and are reasonable choices if it is necessary to prescribe this class of medication when there is hepatic dysfunction.

Sedation and impairment of performance

- Benzodiazepine-induced sedation may be considered either a therapeutic action or a side effect.

- Whether or not sedation is desired, patients must be warned that driving, engaging in dangerous physical activities, and using hazardous machinery should be avoided during the early stages of treatment with benzodiazepines.

Memory impairment

Benzodiazepines are associated with anterograde amnesia, especially when administered intravenously and in high doses.

Dysinhibition and dyscontrol (paradoxical effect)

- Benzodiazepines may occasionally cause paradoxical anger and behavioral disinhibition.
- A history of hostility, impulsivity, or borderline or antisocial personality disorder is a potential predictor of this reaction.
- Some caution should be exercised when these medications are prescribed to patients with a history of poor impulse control and aggression.

Dependence, withdrawal, and rebound effects

- There is a low abuse potential when benzodiazepines are properly prescribed and their use is supervised. However, physical dependence often occurs when they are taken at higher-than-usual doses or for prolonged periods.
- If a benzodiazepine is discontinued precipitously, withdrawal effects (including hyperpyrexia, seizures, psychosis, and even death) may occur.
- Signs and symptoms of withdrawal may include tachycardia, increased blood pressure, muscle cramps, anxiety, insomnia, panic attacks, impairment of memory and concentration, perceptual disturbances, and delirium. In addition, withdrawal-related derealization, hallucinations, and other psychotic symptoms have been reported. These withdrawal symptoms may begin as early as the day after discontinuation of the benzodiazepine, and they may continue for weeks to months.
- Most psychoactive medications should be discontinued gradually. For patients who have been treated with benzodiazepines for longer than 2–3 months, the dose should be decreased by approximately 10% per week.

Overdose

- Benzodiazepines are remarkably safe in overdose.

- Dangerous effects occur when the overdose includes several sedative drugs, especially alcohol, because of synergistic effects at the chloride ion site and resultant membrane hyperpolarization.

- In an emergency setting, the benzodiazepine antagonist flumazenil may be given intravenously to reverse the effects of a potential overdose. However, flumazenil should be used with caution in a mixed overdose situation where TCA is ingested because it may precipitate TCA-induced arrhythmias and seizures that were suppressed by benzodiazepines.

Drug Interactions

- Most sedative drugs, including narcotics and alcohol, potentiate sedative effects.

- Medications that inhibit hepatic CYP 3A3/4 increase blood levels and hence side effects of clonazepam, alprazolam, midazolam, and triazolam.

- Lorazepam, oxazepam, and temazepam are not dependent on hepatic enzymes for metabolism.

Use in Pregnancy

- Anxiolytics should be avoided during pregnancy and breast-feeding when possible.

- There have been concerns that benzodiazepines, when administered during the first trimester of pregnancy, may increase the risk of malformations, particularly cleft palate. Pooled data from cohort studies do not support an increased risk, but data from case-control studies do suggest a risk (Rosenberg et al. 1983).

- Some reports have noted that use of benzodiazepines at close proximity to labor may lead to discontinuation symptoms in the neonate such as hypotonia, apnea, and temperature dysregulation. This risk must be balanced with the risk of worsening of the patient's disorder at time of delivery.

Buspirone

- Buspirone is a partial agonist at 5-HT_{1A} receptors and does not interact with the GABA receptor or the chloride ion channel.
- Buspirone does not produce sedation, interact with alcohol, impair psychomotor performance, or pose a risk of abuse.
- There is no cross-tolerance between benzodiazepines and buspirone, so benzodiazepines cannot be abruptly replaced with buspirone.
- Buspirone cannot be used to treat alcohol or barbiturate withdrawal and detoxification.
- Like the antidepressants, buspirone has a relatively slow onset of action.

INDICATIONS

- Buspirone is effective in the treatment of generalized anxiety. Although the onset of therapeutic action is less rapid, buspirone's efficacy is not statistically different from that of benzodiazepines (Cohn and Wilcox 1986; Goldberg and Finnerty 1979).
- Buspirone does not appear to be effective against panic disorder (Sheehan et al. 1990), although it might reduce anticipatory anxiety.
- Buspirone is also used as an augmenting agent in the treatment of OCD and depression, and there is some evidence that buspirone therapy may be an effective treatment for social phobia.

CLINICAL USE

- The usual initial dosage is 7.5 mg bid, increased after 1 week to 15 mg bid.
- The usual recommended maximum daily dose is 60 mg, but many patients safely tolerate and benefit from dosages up to 90 mg/day.
- Buspirone is metabolized by the liver and excreted by the kidneys, and thus should not be administered to patients with severe hepatic or renal impairment.

SIDE EFFECTS

Side effects include nausea, headache, nervousness, insomnia, dizziness, and light-headedness. Restlessness has also been reported.

Overdose

No fatal outcomes of buspirone overdose have been reported.

Drug Interactions

- Buspirone is metabolized by CYP 3A3/4. Therefore, the initial dose should be lower in patients who are also taking medications known to inhibit these enzymes, such as nefazodone.
- Buspirone should not be administered in combination with an MAOI.

Zolpidem and Zaleplon

- Zolpidem (Ambien) and zaleplon (Sonata) are hypnotics that act at the omega-1 receptor of the central $GABA_A$ receptor complex. This selectivity is hypothesized to be associated with a lower risk of dependence; however, these agents should not be considered free of abuse potential.
- Zolpidem and zaleplon do not appear to have significant anxiolytic, muscle relaxant, or anticonvulsant properties. However, amnestic effects may occur.
- The half-life of zaleplon is 1 hour, and the half-life of zolpidem is 1.5–5 hours.

Indications

- Zolpidem is a short-acting hypnotic with established efficacy in inducing and maintaining sleep. Because of the short half-life, most patients taking zolpidem report minimal daytime sedation.
- Zaleplon is an ultra-short-acting hypnotic and can therefore be administered in the middle of the night. There are minimal residual sedative effects after 4 hours.
- Zaleplon, zolpidem, and a similar selective $GABA_A$ hypnotic, indiplon, have ongoing trials of different modified-release formulations (CR). These versions may help improve the sleep of those patients who have sleep maintenance insomnia or early-morning awakening.

Clinical Use

- Both zolpidem and zaleplon are available in 5- and 10-mg tablets.

- The maximum recommended dosage for adults is 10 mg/day for zolpidem and 20 mg/day for zaleplon, administered at bedtime.
- The initial dose for elderly persons should not exceed 5 mg.
- Caution is advised in patients with hepatic dysfunction.
- In general, hypnotics should be limited to short-term use, with reevaluation for more extended therapy.

SIDE EFFECTS

- In general, side effects are similar to those of short-acting benzodiazepines.

OVERDOSE

- Zolpidem and zaleplon appear to be nonfatal in overdose. However, overdoses in combination with other central nervous system depressant agents pose a greater risk.
- Recommended treatment of overdose consists of general symptomatic and supportive measures, including gastric lavage. Flumazenil may be helpful.

Eszopiclone

- Eszopiclone (Lunesta) is thought to act on GABA receptor complexes close to benzodiazepine receptors.
- No anxiolytic effect has been documented in the literature on this medication.
- The half-life of eszopiclone is approximately 6 hours.

INDICATIONS

- Eszopiclone has established efficacy in inducing and maintaining sleep.
- Its duration of action is approximately 8 hours.

CLINICAL USE

- Eszopiclone is available in 1-, 2-, and 3-mg tablets for oral administration.
- The maximum recommended dosage is 3 mg/night.

- In the elderly the maximum dose is reduced to 2 mg.
- No evidence of tolerance or dependence has been reported, and the FDA has approved this medication for long-term use; however, caution is still advised in long-term use.
- This medication should be used cautiously in patients who abuse alcohol or other drugs because trials of eszopiclone have shown euphoric effects at a high dose.

SIDE EFFECTS

The side effects of eszopiclone are similar to those of short-acting benzodiazepines. Dizziness, headache, and unpleasant taste were the most commonly reported side effects.

OVERDOSE

- No fatalities have been reported with up to 36 mg of eszopiclone being taken in overdose.
- Overdose symptoms include impairment in consciousness, somnolence, and coma.
- Treatment of overdose is symptom driven and supportive. Flumazenil may be beneficial.

DRUG INTERACTIONS

- Eszopiclone is metabolized in the liver by CYP 3A4. It should not be used in patients with severe hepatic impairment.
- Dose adjustment and caution are recommended in patients taking enzyme inhibitors such as ketoconazole, ciprofloxacin, erythromycin, isoniazid, and nefazodone.

Ramelteon

- Ramelteon (Rozerem) is a hypnotic with melatonin receptor agonist activity targeting MT1 and MT2.
- Ramelteon has not been proved to induce dependence.
- As with zolpidem and zaleplon, no known anxiolytic properties have been elicited.
- The half-life of ramelteon is 1–2.6 hours.

INDICATIONS

Ramelteon is indicated for the treatment of insomnia, specifically for improving sleep latency.

CLINICAL USE

- Ramelteon is available in an 8-mg tablet for oral administration.
- The medication should be used with caution in elderly patients because plasma levels in these patients were twice that of healthy adults in clinical trials.
- Ramelteon should not be used by patients with severe hepatic impairment.

SIDE EFFECTS

- The most common side effects of ramelteon are somnolence, dizziness, and fatigue. However, because of its short half-life, this medication is not thought to be associated with daytime sedation.
- Ramelteon is associated with decreased testosterone levels and increased prolactin levels.

OVERDOSE

- Ramelteon appears to be nonfatal in overdose.
- Supportive measures are recommended if overdose occurs. Gastric lavage should be considered.

DRUG INTERACTIONS

- Ramelteon is metabolized hepatically, and CYP 1A2 is the major isozyme involved.
- Caution is recommended with other inhibitory agents such as fluvoxamine.

Stimulants

Stimulants are approved by the FDA for the treatment of ADHD in children and adolescents and for the treatment of narcolepsy; they are also used as augmentation therapy in the treatment of depression. Table 14–13 lists the formulations of the various stimulant medications.

TABLE 14–13. Stimulant medications

DRUG	TRADE NAME	FORMULATIONS
Methylphenidate	Concerta	18-, 27-, 36-, 54-mg extended-release tablets
	Metadate CD	10-, 20-, 30-, 40-, 50-, 60-mg capsules (can be opened and sprinkled over small amount of applesauce before immediate consumption)
	Metadate ER	10-, 20-mg tablets Must be taken whole
	Methylin	5-, 10-, 20-mg tablets
	Methylin Chewable Tablets	2.5-, 5-, 10-mg chewable tablets
	Methylin ER	10-, 20-mg tablets Must be taken whole
	Methylin Oral Solution	5-mg/5-mL, 10-mg/5-mL grape-flavored solutions
	Ritalin	5-, 10-, 20-mg tablets
	Ritalin LA	10-, 20-, 30-, 40-mg extended-release capsules (can be opened and sprinkled over small amount of applesauce before immediate consumption)

TABLE 14–13.   Stimulant medications *(continued)*

DRUG	TRADE NAME	FORMULATIONS
Methylphenidate *(continued)*	Ritalin-SR	20-mg sustained-release tablets Must be taken whole
	Daytrana	10-, 15-, 20-, 30-mg per 9 hour transdermal patches
Dexmethylphenidate	Focalin	2.5-, 5-, 10-mg tablets
	Focalin XR	5-, 10-, 15-, 20-mg extended-release capsules (can be opened and sprinkled over applesauce before immediate consumption)
Dextroamphetamine	DextroStat	5-, 10-mg tablets
	Dexedrine Spansule	5-, 10-, 15-mg sustained-release capsules
Amphetamine/ dextroamphetamine	Adderall	5-, 7.5-, 10-, 12.5-, 15-, 20-, 30-mg tablets
	Adderall XR	5-, 10-, 15-, 20-, 25-, 30-mg extended-release capsules (can be opened and sprinkled on applesauce before immediate consumption)

[a]Because of the risk of hepatic failure, pemoline should not be considered a first-line medication.
Source.   Data from Fuller and Sajatovic 2000; Lee et al. 2003; Pentikis et al. 2002; Physicians' Desk Reference 2007; Tulloch et al. 2002.

Mechanisms of Action

- Stimulants enhance dopamine synaptic transmission (Wilens and Biederman 1992).
- Methylphenidate stimulates the release of dopamine stores from vesicles in presynaptic neurons (Russell et al. 1998), and it may also inhibit presynaptic dopamine reuptake and affect noradrenergic and serotonergic neurotransmission (Challman and Lipsky 2000).
- Dextroamphetamine also has been shown to facilitate the release of dopamine from presynaptic neuron cytoplasmic stores (Masand and Tesar 1996).
- Pemoline blocks presynaptic dopamine reuptake in animals (Homsi et al. 2000).
- The exact mechanisms by which these agents effect their specific actions in treating ADHD have not been definitively established.

Pharmacokinetics

- Stimulants are rapidly absorbed from the gastrointestinal tract with oral administration and are excreted in the urine.
- Stimulants are not highly protein bound.
- Stimulants are lipophilic and thus cross the blood-brain barrier and the placenta.

Table 14–14 summarizes the pharmacokinetic properties and approximate durations of action of stimulants.

Contraindications

- History of hypersensitivity to the particular drug
- Significant cardiovascular disease
- Moderate to severe uncontrolled hypertension
- Hyperthyroidism
- Significant anxiety/agitation
- Glaucoma
- History of drug abuse
- Concomitant use of MAOIs

TABLE 14–14. Pharmacokinetic properties and approximate durations of action of stimulants

Drug	Trade name	Time to peak plasma concentration (hours)	Half-life (mean hours)	Duration of action in ADHD (hours)[a]
Methylphenidate	Concerta	1–2 (initial peak) 6–8 (second peak)	3.5	10–12
	Metadate CD	1.5 (initial peak) 4.5 (second peak)	6.8	8–9
	Metadate ER, Methylin ER, Ritalin-SR	4.7	3–4	6–8
	Methylin, Ritalin	1–2	2–4	4
	Ritalin LA	1–3 (initial peak) 5–11 (second peak)	2.5 (children) 3.5 (adults)	8–9
Dexmethylphenidate	Focalin	1–1.5	2.2	4–6
	Focalin XR	1.5 (initial peak) 6.5 (second peak)	2–3 (children) 2–4.5 (adults)	>6
Dextroamphetamine	Dexedrine Spansule	8	12	6–8
	Dextrostat	2–3	10.5–12	4

TABLE 14–14. Pharmacokinetic properties and approximate durations of action of stimulants *(continued)*

DRUG	TRADE NAME	TIME TO PEAK PLASMA CONCENTRATION (HOURS)	HALF-LIFE (MEAN HOURS)	DURATION OF ACTION IN ADHD (HOURS)[a]
Amphetamine/ dextroamphetamine	Adderall	3	*d*-amphetamine: 9.7-11 *l*-amphetamine: 11-13.8	Dose dependent; 3.5 (5-mg dose) 6.4 (20-mg dose)
	Adderall XR	7	*d*-amphetamine: 10 (adults) 9 (children) *l*-amphetamine: 13 (adults) 11 (children)	10–12
Pemoline	Cylert	2–4	12	6-8

[a]Times are approximate and may vary from patient to patient.

Note. ADHD=attention-deficit/hyperactivity disorder.

Source. Data from L.E. Arnold et al. 2004; Biederman and Faraone 2005; Connor and Steingard 2004; Green 2001; McGough et al. 2005a, 2005b; Pelham et al. 1990; Physicians' Desk Reference 2007; Santosh and Taylor 2000; Swanson et al. 2004; Wigal et al. 2004.

- A history of motor tics or a family history of Tourette's disorder (some children with ADHD may experience new tics or worsening of tics)
- Psychosis

Risks, Side Effects, and Their Management

Table 14–15 lists the potential side effects of stimulants.

- Using the lowest effective dose (Table 14–16), taking the medications with meals, and avoiding doses late in the day are strategies that help minimize side effects. See Table 14–17 for futher details concerning drug delivery systems.
- "Rebound" symptoms, including irritability and hyperactivity, have been described and may occur as plasma concentrations decrease after the last daily dose. Management of rebound symptoms may include using a small dose of medication in the late afternoon or switching to a long-acting preparation.
- Withdrawal symptoms, more commonly seen in individuals who chronically abuse high doses of stimulants, include increased sleep with vivid dreams, increased appetite, fatigue, and drug craving.
- Sudden deaths have occurred with amphetamine use in children with cardiac abnormalities, and clinicians are cautioned against administering amphetamine stimulants to patients with structural cardiac abnormalities.

Monitoring Guidelines

- Blood pressure, pulse, height, weight, and appetite should be evaluated, and growth charts should be maintained at baseline and throughout treatment (Greenhill et al. 2002; Santosh and Taylor 2000).
- The patient should also be evaluated for the onset or exacerbation of tics or dyskinesias.
- Because thrombocytopenic purpura and leukopenia can occur, a CBC should be performed periodically.
- Pemoline may affect liver function tests. Discontinue pemoline if the ALT level increases to more than two times the normal level.

TABLE 14–15.　Potential side effects of stimulants

General

Delayed growth	Sweating

HEENT

Headache	Blurred vision

Cardiovascular

Tachycardia	Hypotension
Bradycardia	Chest pain
Hypertension	Palpitations

Gastrointestinal

Nausea	Decreased appetite
Vomiting	Weight loss
Dry mouth	Abdominal pain

Dermatological

Rash	Pruritis

Neurological

Nervousness	Dizziness
Insomnia	Tics
Movement disorders	Tremor
Restlessness	Euphoria
Anxiety	Dysphoria
Agitation	Psychosis
Drowsiness	Seizures
Tourette's disorder	Neuroleptic malignant syndrome

Note.　HEENT=head, ears, eyes, nose, and throat.
Source.　Data from Fuller and Sajatovic 2000; Lee et al. 2003; Pentikis et al. 2002; Physicians' Desk Reference 2007.

TABLE 14–16.   Dosing strategies for stimulants

DRUG	TRADE NAME	GENERAL DOSING STRATEGIES
Methylphenidate	Concerta	ADHD
		Patients ≥6 years old: Start at 18 mg qam; increase by 18 mg/day at weekly intervals
		Maximum daily dose: 54 mg/day
		Switching from other methylphenidate preparations:
		• Start Concerta at 18 mg qam if administering methylphenidate 5 mg bid or tid or SR methylphenidate 20 mg/day.
		• Start Concerta at 36 mg qam if administering methylphenidate 10 mg bid or tid or SR methylphenidate 40 mg/day.
		• Start Concerta at 54 mg qam if administering methylphenidate 15 mg bid or tid or SR methylphenidate 60 mg/day.
		Maximum daily dose: 54 mg (some adolescents may be titrated to a maximum of 72 mg/day, not to exceed 2 mg/kg body weight/day)
		Must be taken whole
	Metadate CD	ADHD: Patients ≥6 years old: Start at 20 mg qam; increase by 10–20 mg/day at weekly intervals as needed to attain response. Maximum daily dose: 60 mg

TABLE 14–16. Dosing strategies for stimulants *(continued)*

DRUG	TRADE NAME	GENERAL DOSING STRATEGIES
Methylphenidate *(continued)*	Metadate ER, Methylin ER, Ritalin-SR,	ADHD: May be given once every morning in place of total daily dose of immediate-release (IR) methylphenidate to achieve an estimated 8-hour duration of action. Must be taken whole.
	Methylin, Ritalin	ADHD and narcolepsy
		Children ≥6 years old: Start at 5 mg qam or bid; increase by 5–10 mg/day at weekly intervals as needed to attain response. Give three times daily if effect is needed in evening hours.
		Adults: Start at 5–10 mg bid; titrate as above.
		Maximum daily dose: 60 mg
	Ritalin LA	ADHD
		Children ≥6 years old: Start at 20 mg once daily (or lower at clinician's discretion); increase by 10 mg weekly.
		Switching from IR or sustained-release (SR) methylphenidate: Start Ritalin LA at total daily dose of IR or SR methylphenidate (administer Ritalin LA dose once daily).
		Maximum daily dose: 60 mg

TABLE 14–16. Dosing strategies for stimulants *(continued)*

Drug	Trade name	General dosing strategies
Dexmethylphenidate	Focalin	ADHD Patients ≥6 years old: Start at 2.5 mg bid; increase by 2.5–5 mg/day at weekly intervals. Switching from IR methylphenidate: Start Focalin at 50% of the methylphenidate dose (administer Focalin in divided twice-daily doses); titrate as above. Maximum daily dose: 10 mg bid
	Focalin XR	ADHD Children ≥6 years old: Start at 5 mg qd; increase by 5 mg/day at weekly intervals. Adults: Start at 10 mg qd; increase by 10 mg/day at weekly intervals. Switching from methylphenidate: Start Focalin XR at 50% of the total daily dose of methylphenidate (administer Focalin XR in a once-daily dose); titrate Focalin XR as above. Switching from IR dexmethylphenidate (Focalin): Start Focalin XR at the same total daily dose of Focalin. Maximum daily dose: 20 mg/day (children and adults)

TABLE 14–16. Dosing strategies for stimulants *(continued)*

DRUG	TRADE NAME	GENERAL DOSING STRATEGIES
Dextroamphetamine	Dexedrine Spansule	ADHD and narcolepsy
		Dosing similar to Dexedrine dosing, except use once-daily dosing when appropriate
	DextroStat	ADHD
		Patients ≥6 years old: Start at 5 mg qam or bid; increase by 5 mg/day at weekly intervals.
		Maximum daily dose: 40 mg
		Narcolepsy
		Children 6–12 years old: Start at 5 mg/day; increase by 5 mg/day at weekly intervals.
		Patients >12 years old: Start at 10 mg/day; increase by 10 mg/day at weekly intervals.
		Maximum daily dose: 60 mg

TABLE 14–16.   Dosing strategies for stimulants *(continued)*

DRUG	TRADE NAME	GENERAL DOSING STRATEGIES
Amphetamine/ dextroamphetamine	Adderall	ADHD
		Children ≥6 years old: Start at 5 mg qam or bid; increase by 5 mg/day at weekly intervals.
		Maximum daily dose: 40 mg
		Narcolepsy
		Children 6–12 years old: Start at 5 mg/day; increase by 5 mg/day at weekly intervals
		Patients >12 years old: Start at 10 mg/day; increase by 10 mg/day at weekly intervals.
		Maximum daily dose: 60 mg
	Adderall XR	ADHD
		Children ≥6 years old: Start at 10 mg qam; increase by 5–10 mg/day at weekly intervals.
		Adults: Recommended dose is 20 mg/day
		Maximum daily dose: 30 mg

TABLE 14–16. Dosing strategies for stimulants *(continued)*

DRUG	TRADE NAME	GENERAL DOSING STRATEGIES
Amphetamine/ dextroamphetamine *(continued)*		Switching from IR Adderall: Switch to the same total daily dose (administer Adderall XR once daily).
		Not studied in children <6 years old
Pemoline	Cylert	ADHD
		Patients >6 years old: Start at 37.5 mg qam; increase by 18.75 mg/day at weekly intervals.
		Maximum daily dose: 112.5 mg
		Measure liver transaminase levels before treatment and then every 2 weeks; discontinue pemoline if ALT level increases to more than two times normal.
		Should not be considered first-line agent (risk of hepatic failure)
		Obtain written informed consent prior to initiation of treatment.

Note. ADHD=attention-deficit/hyperactivity disorder; ALT=alanine transaminase; bid=twice a day; qam=every morning; qd=each day; tid=three times a day.

Source. Fuller and Sajatovic 2000; Physicians' Desk Reference 2007; Spencer et al. 2003.

TABLE 14–17. Drug delivery systems of long-acting stimulant formulations

DRUG	TRADE NAME	DRUG DELIVERY SYSTEM
Methylphenidate	Concerta	Tablet that contains approximately 22% of methylphenidate dose in an IR capsule overcoat, and 78% within the tablet that is released by an osmotic process over an extended period of time
	Metadate CD	Capsules that provide 30% of methylphenidate dose by IR beads and 70% of the dose by extended-release beads
	Metadate ER	Slowly absorbed tablet
	Ritalin LA	Capsule with 50% methylphenidate dose as immediate-release (IR) beads and 50% as delayed-release beads
	Ritalin-SR	Slowly absorbed tablet
Dexmethylphenidate	Focalin XR	Capsules with 50% dexmethylphenidate dose as IR beads and 50% as delayed-release beads
Dextroamphetamine	Dexedrine Spansule	Capsule that allows some medication to be released immediately and the remainder to be released over time
Amphetamine/ dextroamphetamine	Adderall XR	Capsules with one bead type providing an immediate release of medication and another bead type releasing medication 4–6 hours after administration

Source. Connor and Steingard 2004; Physicians' Desk Reference 2007.

Overdose

- Symptoms of stimulant overdose include tremors, hypertension, fever, tachycardia, hyperreflexia, confusion, agitation, and psychosis.

- Management of overdose includes stopping the medication and supportive treatment.

Methylphenidate

- Methylphenidate is structurally similar to amphetamine.

- This medication is available in immediate-release, extended-release, and controlled-release formulations. The immediate-release formulation has a very short half-life, reaches peak plasma concentrations in 1–2 hours, and thus is dosed multiple times per day.

- Methylphenidate is hepatically metabolized to an inactive metabolite and excreted by the kidneys.

ADVERSE REACTIONS

- Methylphenidate may decrease therapeutic effects of concomitantly administered antihypertensive medications and may potentiate effects of warfarin, phenytoin, phenylbutazone, and TCAs.

- When methylphenidate and MAOIs are coadministered, hypertensive crisis may result.

Dextroamphetamine

- Dextroamphetamine is the *d*-isomer of amphetamine.

- This medication is available in immediate-release and extended-release formulations.

- Dextroamphetamine is functionally more potent than methylphenidate and may be associated with a greater risk of growth retardation and abuse.

- The dextroamphetamine/amphetamine combination Adderall is also more potent than methylphenidate, and it has a longer half-life.

- Adderall XR, an extended-release formulation, reaches peak plasma concentrations in 7 hours and has a half-life of approximately 9–11 hours in children and 10–13 hours in adults. This long-acting formulation is bioequivalent to a similar total dose of Adderall administered twice daily (Tulloch et al. 2002) and may provide therapeutic effects in ADHD over a 12-hour period (Biederman et al. 2002; McCracken et al. 2003).

ADVERSE REACTIONS

- The risk of tachycardia, hypertension, and cardiotoxicity is increased with coadministration of dronabinol and dextroamphetamine.
- Administration of dextroamphetamine with MAOIs may increase the risk of hypertensive crisis.
- Alkalinizing agents can speed absorption or delay urinary excretion of dextroamphetamine.
- Gastric or urinary acidifying agents can decrease the effects of dextroamphetamine.
- Propoxyphene overdose can potentiate amphetamine central nervous system stimulation, potentially resulting in fatal convulsions.

Pemoline

- Has a long half-life, allowing for once-daily dosing
- Has fewer stimulating properties than other stimulants and may have less abuse potential
- Does not require triplicate prescriptions
- Therapeutic action in ADHD occurs by week 3 or 4
- Numerous reports of hepatotoxicity in patients taking pemoline and therefore not a first-line agent
- Serum hepatic transaminase levels should be determined at baseline and then every 2 weeks
- Should be discontinued if serum alanine transaminase levels increase to two times the upper limit of normal

Modafinil

- Modafinil (Provigil) was approved to improve wakefulness in patients with narcolepsy, obstructive sleep apnea/hypopnea syndrome (as an adjunct to standard treatments for the underlying disorder), and shift work sleep disorder.

- Modafinil has a long duration of action and low potential for dependence and may be a reasonable first choice in the treatment of mild to moderate narcolepsy (Silber 2001).
- This medication does not require a triplicate prescription.
- The mechanism of action for modafinil is unclear but is thought to differ from that of conventional stimulants.
- Modafinil is metabolized by the liver and excreted by the kidneys.
- The half-life of this drug is approximately 15 hours.
- Modafinil can decrease the serum levels and effectiveness of oral contraceptives.

Nonstimulant Medication for ADHD: Atomoxetine

Atomoxetine (Strattera) is a nonstimulant medication. It is especially useful for patients with ADHD who have not done well on stimulants because of poor efficacy or tolerability, as well as for patients in whom the abuse potential of stimulants is of particular concern.

- Atomoxetine is available in 10-, 18-, 25-, 40-, 60-, 80-, and 100-mg capsules.
- In children and adolescents who weigh less than 70 kg, start at a total daily dose of 0.5 mg/kg body weight and increase after a minimum of 3 days to a target daily dose of 1.2 mg/kg (either as a single morning dose or divided evenly into morning and late afternoon doses), not to exceed a total daily dose of the lesser of 1.4 mg/kg body weight or 100 mg. In patients weighing more than 70 kg, start at a total daily dose of 40 mg and increase after a minimum of 3 days to a total daily dose of 80 mg. If needed, the dose may be increased to 100 mg.
- This drug is highly protein bound and reaches peak plasma concentrations in 1–2 hours.
- Atomoxetine is a selective inhibitor of norepinephrine presynaptic reuptake transporters that has been shown to increase extracellular norepinephrine and dopamine concentrations in the prefrontal cortex in rats (Bymaster et al. 2002).
- This medication is contraindicated in patients with narrow-angle glaucoma or in combination with an MAOI.

- Children and adolescents taking atomoxetine should be monitored for the appearance or worsening of aggressive or hostile behavior.

Side Effects

- Common side effects include headache, upper abdominal pain, decreased appetite, nausea, vomiting, irritability, and dizziness (Wernicke and Kratochvil 2002). Other side effects observed in clinical trials of adults include constipation, somnolence, dry mouth, insomnia, urinary hesitancy and/or retention, and impaired sexual function.
- Postmarketing reports suggest severe liver injury in rare cases.
- Atomoxetine may increase heart rate and blood pressure, and it should be used with caution in patients with hypertension, tachycardia, cardiovascular disease, or cerebrovascular disease. Orthostatic hypotension has also been reported.

Drug Interactions

- Paroxetine, a potent CYP 2D6 inhibitor, has been shown to increase plasma concentrations of atomoxetine and significantly increase the half-life of atomoxetine approximately 2.5-fold in patients who are extensive 2D6 metabolizers.
- Atomoxetine may potentiate the cardiovascular effects of albuterol or other pressor agents.

Cognitive Enhancers

This section describes two classes of pharmacological agents used in the treatment of Alzheimer's disease: the cholinesterase inhibitors and the N-methyl-D-aspartate (NMDA) receptor antagonists.

Cholinesterase Inhibitors

The cholinesterase inhibitors include donepezil, galantamine, rivastigmine, and tacrine. The cholinesterase inhibitors cross the blood-brain barrier and decrease enzymatic hydrolysis of acetylcholine in the synaptic cleft, thereby increasing acetylcholine availability for neurotransmission.

Table 14–18 summarizes dosing guidelines and available formulations, and Table 14–19 summarizes the pharmacokinetics and key features of these drugs.

CLINICAL USE

- Treatment should be considered as early as possible after patients have been diagnosed with Alzheimer's disease.
- Donepezil, galantamine, and rivastigmine can each be considered a reasonable first-choice medication.
- The optimal duration of treatment with cholinesterase inhibitors has not been definitely established.
  - Most randomized, controlled trials in patients with mild to moderate Alzheimer's disease have been 26 weeks or less in duration.
  - Some data suggest continued benefits with treatment for 1 year or longer.

- If a patient has an inadequate treatment response to one cholinesterase inhibitor, he or she may benefit from a trial of a different agent within the class.
- Although clinicians often use each cholinesterase inhibitor in combination with memantine, the best evidence to date for such combination treatment is the use of memantine in patients with moderate to severe Alzheimer's disease already taking donepezil (Tariot et al. 2004).

SIDE EFFECTS

- Common side effects include nausea, vomiting, abdominal pain, diarrhea, and dizziness. These side effects tend to be associated with treatment initiation or early dose increases and are often transient.
- Anorexia and weight loss may also occur and may persist throughout treatment.
- Potentially dangerous side effects include myasthenia, respiratory depression, and bradycardia.
- Use these medications with caution in patients with cardiac conduction problems, because vagotonic effects can lead to bradycardia.

TABLE 14–18.　Cholinesterase inhibitors available in the United States

DRUG	TRADE NAME	DOSING GUIDELINES	FORMULATIONS
Donepezil	Aricept	Administer 5 mg po qhs (with or without a meal) for 4–6 weeks. Some patients then increase to 10 mg/day if tolerated. Target daily dosage range: 5–10 mg po qhs	5-, 10-mg tablets 5-, 10-mg oral disintegrating tablets (Aricept ODT) 1 mg/mL oral solution
Galantamine	Razadyne	Administer 4 mg po bid (preferably with meals) for at least 4 weeks, then increase to an initial target dosage of 8 mg bid for at least 4 weeks. A further dosage increase to 12 mg bid may be helpful for some patients. Target daily dosage range: 8–12 mg po bid	4-, 8-, 12-mg tablets 4-mg/mL oral solution (in 100-mL bottle with calibrated pipette)
	Razadyne ER	Administer 8 mg po qam (preferably with meal) for at least 4 weeks, then increase to an initial target dosage of 16 mg po qam. A further dosage increase to 24 mg po qam may be helpful for some patients. Target daily dosage range: 16–24 mg po qam	8-, 16-, 24-mg capsules

TABLE 14–18. Cholinesterase inhibitors available in the United States

DRUG	TRADE NAME	DOSING GUIDELINES	FORMULATIONS
Rivastigmine	Exelon	Administer 1.5 mg po bid (preferably with meals) for 2–4 weeks, then increase in increments of 1.5 mg/dose every 2–4 weeks, as tolerated, to a maximum dosage of 6 mg po bid. Target daily dosage range: 3–6 mg po bid	1.5-, 3-, 4.5-, 6-mg capsules 2-mg/mL oral solution (in bottles of 120-mL with dosing syringe)
	Exelon Patch	Administer 4.6-mg/24-hour dosage for a minimum of 4 weeks, then increase to 9.5-mg/24-hour dosage	4.6- and 9.5-mg/24-hour patches
Tacrine	Cognex	Administer 10 mg po qid for 4 weeks, then 20 mg qid for 4 weeks, then 30 mg qid for 4 weeks, and then 40 mg qid. Titration is based on tolerability and serum transaminase levels. Refer to current product labeling for guidelines on dose adjustments, monitoring, and rechallenging.	10-, 20-, 30-, 40-mg capsules

Note. bid=twice a day; po=orally; qam=every morning; qd=each day; qhs=every bedtime; qid=four times a day.
Source. Doody et al. 2001; Physicians' Desk Reference 2007; Schneider 2001.

TABLE 14–19. Pharmacokinetics and key features of cholinesterase inhibitors

AGENT	PROTEIN BINDING	HALF-LIFE (HOURS)	RELATIONS TO CYTOCHROME P450 (CYP) SYSTEM	OTHER KEY FEATURES
Donepezil (Aricept)	>95%	70	CYP 2D6 substrate CYP 3A4 substrate	Once-daily dosing
Galantamine (Razadyne, Razadyne ER)	18%	7	CYP 2D6 substrate CYP 3A4 substrate	Allosteric nicotinic receptor activity Once-daily dosing for ER formulation
Rivastigmine (Exelon)	40%	1.5	None anticipated	Not hepatically metabolized (metabolized by hydrolysis and renally eliminated) Dual acetylcholinesterase and butyrylcholinesterase inhibitor
Tacrine (Cognex)	55%	24	CYP 1A2 substrate CYP 1A2 inhibitor	Risk for hepatotoxicity Multiple doses daily Requires close hepatic monitoring

Source.   Bores et al. 1996; Fuller and Sajatovic 2000; Physicians' Desk Reference 2007; Watkins et al. 1994.

- Caution is warranted in patients with comorbid asthma, chronic obstructive pulmonary disease, bladder outlet obstruction, or seizures, as well as in patients at risk for gastrointestinal ulcers or bleeding (Fuller and Sajatovic 2000).

DRUG INTERACTIONS

- All cholinesterase inhibitors can exaggerate the effects of succinylcholine-like muscle relaxants during anesthesia.
- Use of cholinesterase inhibitors in combination with other cholinergic agents, such as bethanechol, can lead to synergistic effects and increased toxicity.
- Concomitant use of anticholinergic agents and cholinesterase inhibitors can decrease the effectiveness of both agents.

DONEPEZIL

- Donepezil is a selective, reversible inhibitor of acetylcholinesterase.
- Its long half-life allows for once-daily dosing.
- Although donepezil is currently only approved by the FDA for the treatment of mild to moderate Alzheimer's disease, its efficacy has also been examined in other dementias, including moderate to severe Alzheimer's disease, Parkinson's disease, and vascular dementia.

Side effects

- Common side effects include nausea, vomiting, diarrhea, abdominal pain, anorexia, weight loss, insomnia, and fatigue.
- Some patients may also experience muscle cramps, dizziness, and syncope.

GALANTAMINE

Galantamine is a competitive, reversible cholinesterase inhibitor and an allosteric modulator of presynaptic nicotinic receptors, thereby enhancing synaptic acetylcholine activity.

Side effects

- Common side effects reported in clinical trials include nausea, vomiting, diarrhea, anorexia, weight loss, dizziness, abdominal pain, and tremor.

- Most side effects tend to be dose related and may be decreased with a slow titration schedule of 4 mg bid every 4 weeks.

RIVASTIGMINE

- Rivastigmine is a reversible acetylcholinesterase inhibitor that is relatively selective for an acetylcholinesterase subtype found on postsynaptic membranes. It is also an inhibitor of butyrylcholinesterase, which is largely of glial origin.
- Rivastigmine is not hepatically metabolized; however, the pharmacodynamic interactions (noted earlier in this chapter) associated with other cholinesterase inhibitors may occur.

Side effects

- Common side effects include nausea, vomiting, and weight loss, especially with high-dose treatment.
- Recent data suggest that side effects may be decreased by titrating no faster than 1.5 mg bid every 2 weeks (Vellas et al. 1998).
- Severe vomiting may occur if rivastigmine therapy is resumed after a treatment interruption.

TACRINE

Tacrine was the first cholinesterase inhibitor to be approved by the FDA for the treatment of mild to moderate dementia.

- Tacrine is not considered first-line, and it is rarely used because of the risk of hepatotoxicity.
- Serum transaminase levels must be monitored every 2 weeks from at least week 4 to week 16 after initiation of tacrine treatment.
- In controlled trials of tacrine for the treatment of dementia, up to 50% of patients taking high-dose tacrine had increased transaminase levels (see review by Doody et al. 2001), and 25% had increases in ALT concentrations beyond three times the upper limit of normal.

NMDA Receptor Antagonists

Memantine, an NMDA receptor antagonist, is the only medication approved by the FDA for the treatment of moderate to severe dementia of the Alzheimer's type.

- Memantine is available in 5- and 10-mg tablets, and also in oral solution (2mg/mL).

- The typical starting dose is 5 mg as a single daily dose. Subsequent dose increases should occur in 5-mg increments (at least 1 week apart) to a target dosage of 10 mg twice daily (or 5 mg twice daily in patients with renal impairment).

- Memantine is a moderate-affinity, noncompetitive inhibitor of NMDA receptors.

- Memantine is not highly protein bound, and it has a half-life of 60–80 hours.

- It is primarily renally excreted unchanged in the urine; however, a portion of the administered dose is converted to three inactive metabolites. Clinicians are advised to use lower doses in patients with renal impairment and to avoid use in patients with severe renal impairment.

- The most common side effects of memantine are dizziness, headache, confusion, constipation, coughing, hypertension, somnolence, pain, vomiting, and hallucinations.

DRUG INTERACTIONS

- Memantine is not a major substrate for hepatic CYP isoenzymes and has not been shown to significantly inhibit or induce these enzymes.

- Concomitant use of another medication that uses the same renal system (e.g., triamterene, hydrochlorothiazide, digoxin, cimetidine, ranitidine, metformin, and quinidine) may affect plasma levels of both drugs.

- Memantine should be not be used in combination with other NMDA receptor antagonists, such as amantadine or dextromethorphan, because these combinations have not been formally studied.

- The clearance of memantine can be reduced when the urine is alkalinized, such as with the concomitant use of sodium bicarbonate or carbonic anhydrase inhibitors, or during severe urinary tract infections.

References

Arnold LE, Lindsay RL, Connors CK, et al: A double-blind, placebo-controlled withdrawal trial of dexmethylphenidate hydrochloride in children with attention-deficit hyperactivity disorder. J Am Acad Child Adolesc Psychiatry 14:542–554, 2004

Arnold LM, Lu Y, Crofford LJ, et al: A double-blind, multicenter trial comparing duloxetine with placebo in the treatment of fibromyalgia patients with or without major depressive disorder. Arthritis Rheum 50:2974–2984, 2004

Biederman J, Faraone SV: Attention-deficit hyperactivity disorder. Lancet 366:237–248, 2005

Biederman J, Lopez FA, Boellner SW, et al: A randomized, double-blind, placebo-controlled, parallel-group study of SLI381 (Adderall XR) in children with attention-deficit/hyperactivity disorder. Pediatrics 110:258–266, 2002

Bores GM, Huger FP, Petko W, et al: Pharmacological evaluation of novel Alzheimer's disease therapeutics: acetylcholinesterase inhibitors related to galanthamine. J Pharmacol Exp Ther 277:728–738, 1996

Bymaster FP, Katner JS, Nelson DL, et al: Atomoxetine increases extracellular levels of norepinephrine and dopamine in prefrontal cortex of rat: a potential mechanism for efficacy in attention-deficit/hyperactivity disorder. Neuropsychopharmacology 27:699–711, 2002

Challman TD, Lipsky JJ: Methylphenidate: its pharmacology and uses. Mayo Clin Proc 75:711–721, 2000

Cohn JB, Wilcox CS: Low-sedation potential of buspirone compared with alprazolam and lorazepam in the treatment of anxious patients: a double-blind study. J Clin Psychiatry 47:409–412, 1986

Connor DF, Steingard RJ: New formulations of stimulants for attention deficit hyperactivity disorder: therapeutic potential. CNS Drugs14:1011–1030, 2004

Cummings JL, Trimble MR: Concise Guide to Neuropsychiatry and Behavioral Neurology, 2nd Edition. Washington, DC, American Psychiatric Publishing, 2002

Doody RS, Geldmacher DS, Gordon B, et al: Open-label, multi-center, phase 3 extension study of the safety and efficacy of donepezil in patients with Alzheimer disease. Arch Neurol 58:427–433, 2001

Ereshefsky L, Toney G, Saklad SR, et al: A loading-dose strategy for converting from oral to depot haloperidol. Hosp Community Psychiatry 44:1155–1161, 1993

Fuller MA, Sajatovic M: Psychotropic Drug Information Handbook. Hudson, OH, Lexi-Comp, 2000

Gardner DM, Lynd LD: Sumatriptan contraindications and the serotonin syndrome. Ann Pharmacother 32:33–38, 1998

Goldberg HL, Finnerty RJ: The comparative efficacy of buspirone and diazepam in the treatment of anxiety. Am J Psychiatry 136:1184–1187, 1979

Green WH: Child and Adolescent Clinical Psychopharmacology, 3rd Edition. Philadelphia, PA, Lippincott Williams & Wilkins, 2001

Greenhill LL, Pliszka S, Dulcan MK, et al: Practice parameters for the use of stimulant medications in the treatment of children, adolescents, and adults. J Am Acad Child Adolesc Psychiatry 41(suppl 2):26s–49s, 2002

Herrmann N, Lanctôt KL: Do atypical antipsychotics cause stroke? CNS Drugs 19:91–103, 2005

Holmes LB, Baldwin EJ, Smith CR, et al: Increased frequency of isolated cleft palate in infants exposed to lamotrigine during pregnancy. Neurology 70:2152–2158, 2008

Homsi J, Walsh D, Nelson KA: Psychostimulants in supportive care. Support Care Cancer 8:385–397, 2000

Jenike MA: Affective illness in elderly patients, part 2. Psychiatric Times 4:1, 1987

Ketter TA, Wang PW, Chandler RA, et al: Dermatology precautions and slower titration yield low incidence of lamotrigine treatment-emergent rash. J Clin Psychiatry 66(5):642–645, 2005

Kilian JG, Kerr K, Lawrence C, et al: Myocarditis and cardiomyopathy associated with clozapine. Lancet 354:1841–1845, 1999

Lamictal [package insert]. Research Triangle Park, GlaxoSmithKline, 2005

Lee L, Kepple J, Wang Y, et al: Bioavailability of modified-release methylphenidate: influence of high-fat breakfast when administered intact and when capsule content sprinkled on applesauce. Biopharm Drug Dispos 24:233–243, 2003

Liebowitz MR, Quitkin FM, Stewart JW, et al: Phenelzine v imipramine in atypical depression: a preliminary report. Arch Gen Psychiatry 41:669–677, 1984

Masand PS, Tesar GE: Use of stimulants in the medically ill. Psychiatr Clin North Am 19:515–547, 1996

McCracken JT, Biederman J, Greenhill LL, et al: Analog classroom assessment of a once-daily mixed amphetamine formulation, SLI381 (Adderall XR), in children with ADHD. J Am Acad Child Adolesc Psychiatry 42:673–683, 2003

McGough JJ, Biederman J, Wigal SB, et al: Long-term tolerability and effectiveness of once daily mixed amphetamine salts (Adderall XR) in children with ADHD. J Am Acad Child Adolesc Psychiatry 44:530–538, 2005a

McGough JJ, Pataki CS, Suddath R: Dexmethylphenidate extended-release capsules for attention deficit hyperactivity disorder. Expert Rev Neurother 5:437–441, 2005b

Oldham JM: Guideline Watch: Practice Guidelines for the Treatment of Patients With Borderline Personality Disorder. Arlington, VA, American Psychiatric Association, 2005

Pelham WE Jr, Greenslade KE, Vodde-Hamilton M, et al: Relative efficacy of long acting stimulants on children with attention deficit-hyperactivity disorder: a comparison of standard methylphenidate, sustained-release methylphenidate, sustained-release dextroamphetamine, and pemoline. Pediatrics 86:226–237, 1990

Pentikis HS, Simmons RD, Benedict MF, et al: Methylphenidate bioavailability in adults when an extended-release multiparticulate formulation is administered sprinkled on food or as an intact capsule. J Am Acad Child Adolesc Psychiatry 41:443–449, 2002

Physicians' Desk Reference, 61st Edition. Montvale, NJ, Thompson PDR, 2007

Quitkin FM, Rifkin A, Klein DF: Monoamine oxidase inhibitors: a review of antidepressant effectiveness. Arch Gen Psychiatry 36:749–760, 1979

Ravaris CL, Robinson DS, Ives JO, et al: Phenelzine and amitriptyline in the treatment of depression: a comparison of present and past studies. Arch Gen Psychiatry 37:1075–1080, 1980

Rosenberg L, Mitchell AA, Parsells JL, et al: Lack of relation of oral clefts to diazepam use during pregnancy. N Engl J Med 309:1282–1285, 1983

Russell V, de Villiers A, Sagvolden T, et al: Differences between electrically-, Ritalin- and D-amphetamine-stimulated release of [3H]dopamine from brain slices suggest impaired vesicular storage of dopamine in an animal model of attention-deficit hyperactivity disorder. Behav Brain Res 94:163–171, 1998

Santosh PJ, Taylor E: Stimulant drugs. Eur Child Adolesc Psychiatry 9 (suppl 1):I27–I43, 2000

Schneider LS: Treatment of Alzheimer's disease with cholinesterase inhibitors. Clin Geriatr Med 17:337–358, 2001

Sheehan DV, Raj AB, Sheehan KH, et al: Is buspirone effective for panic disorder? J Clin Psychopharmacol 10:3–11, 1990

Silber MH: Sleep disorders. Neurol Clin 19:173–186, 2001

Spencer T, Greenhill L, on behalf of the Adolescent Study Group: OROS methylphenidate for the treatment of adolescent attention deficit/hyperactivity disorder. Poster presented at the American Academy of Child and Adolescent Psychiatry Annual Meeting, Miami, Florida, October 14–19, 2003

Swanson JM, Wigal SB, Wigal T, et al: A comparison of once-daily extended-release methylphenidate formulations in children with attention-deficit/hyperactivity disorder in the laboratory school (the COMACS Study). Pediatrics 113:e206–e216, 2004

Tariot PN, Farlow MR, Grossberg GT, et al: Memantine treatment in patients with moderate to severe Alzheimer disease already receiving donepezil: a randomized controlled trial. JAMA 291:317–324, 2004

Teboul E, Chouinard G: A guide to benzodiazepine selection, part 1: pharmacological aspects. Can J Psychiatry 35:700–710, 1990

Tulloch SJ, Zhang Y, McLean A, et al: SLI381 (Adderall XR), a two-component, extended release formulation of mixed amphetamine salts: bioavailability of three test formulations and comparison of fasted, fed, and sprinkled administration. Pharmacotherapy 22:1405–1415, 2002

Vellas B, Inglis F, Potkin S: Interim results from an international clinical trial with rivastigmine evaluating a 2-week titration rate in mild to severe Alzheimer's patients. Int J Geriatr Psychopharmacol 1:140–144, 1998

Watkins PB, Zimmerman HJ, Knapp MJ, et al: Hepatotoxic effects of tacrine administration in patients with Alzheimer's disease. JAMA 271:992–998, 1994

Wernicke JF, Kratochvil CJ: Safety profile of atomoxetine in the treatment of children and adolescents with ADHD. J Clin Psychiatry 63 (suppl 12):50–55, 2002

Wigal S, Swanson JM, Feifel D, et al: A double-blind, placebo-controlled trial of dexmethylphenidate hydrochloride and d,l-threo-methylphenidate hydrochloride in children with attention-deficit/hyperactivity disorder. J Am Acad Child Adolesc Psychiatry 43:1406–1414, 2004

Wilens TE, Biederman J: The stimulants. Psychiatr Clin North Am 15:191–222, 1992

Zisook S: A clinical overview of monoamine oxidase inhibitors. Psychosomatics 26:240–246, 1985

15

Psychotherapy and Psychosocial Treatments

Psychoanalysis and Psychodynamic Psychotherapy

Psychoanalysis is a family of psychological theories and methods based on the work of Sigmund Freud and his successors (e.g., Klein, Kohut). As a therapy, psychoanalysis is based on the observation that individuals are often unaware of many of the factors that determine their emotions and behavior. These unconscious factors may create unhappiness, sometimes in the form of recognizable symptoms or in the form of troubling personality traits, difficulties in relationships, or disturbances in self-esteem.

In psychoanalytic theory, the unconscious is a depository for socially unacceptable ideas, wishes or desires, traumatic memories, and painful emotions that are kept from awareness by defense mechanisms (see Table 15–1). Psychoanalytic treatment attempts to gradually trace symptoms (e.g., anxiety or chronic relationship difficulties) back to their once-unconscious origin, typically in childhood. In traditional forms of psychoanalysis, the analyst (therapist/doctor) sits behind as the patient is lying down on a couch. This is so that the analyst can be a blank slate onto which the patient will unconsciously transfer emotions felt toward important people in his or her life. The therapy involves analyzing this transference. Over time, the patient may express feelings toward the doctor that are similar to those felt toward other important people in the

TABLE 15–1. Classic defense mechanisms

Repression	Keeping unwanted affects, memories, and drives from consciousness, allowing them to remain in our behavior outside of awareness. This is the mechanism by which we "forget" unpleasant information or feelings.
Regression	Returning to an earlier level of maturational functioning
Isolation	Separating link between affect and memory. This mechanism is often used by patients with obsessive-compulsive features or disorder.
Reaction formation	Transforming affects into their opposites (e.g., "I don't love this; I hate it"). This mechanism is often used by patients with obsessive-compulsive features or disorder.
Undoing	Attempting to nullify or atone for forbidden fantasy, affect, or memory. This mechanism is used by patients with obsessive-compulsive features or disorder.
Projection	Sending an unacceptable thought or feeling away and attributing it to an external source (e.g., "I don't hate him; he hates me"). Often used by patients with paranoid personality structures or disorders. Projective identification is a more primitive version of this defense mechanism, in which identity is ascribed to another, generally in a relationship in which the other accepts the projection.
Identification	Taking attributes of important others into our own selves, which we can then modify. This defense mechanism can be either part of normal growth or pathological, depending on maturational level.
Turning against	Taking an impulse intended to be expressed toward someone else and directing it against oneself (e.g., biting your tongue by "accident" when you feel like saying something hostile toward another person)

TABLE 15–1. Classic defense mechanisms *(continued)*

Reversal	Taking an impulse and reversing its polarity (e.g., changing sadistic feelings into masochistic ones or transforming the active role into the passive role)
Denial	Invalidating an unpleasant or unwanted piece of information and living life as though it did not exist, such as patients with addictions who do not acknowledge the consequences of their behavior. This mechanism differs from repression in that there is slight consciousness, but a piece of reality is being denied, not just mental content.
Splitting	Keeping "good objects," pleasurable affects, and good memories apart from "bad objects," unpleasurable affects, and bad memories. Early in life, this defense keeps infants from having good experiences drowned out by bad ones. Later, it prevents people from experiencing others as multifaceted, complex whole objects possessing both good and bad characteristics. This is often seen in patients with borderline personality disorder.
Sublimation	Turning drives, affects, and memories into healthy and creative outcomes

Source. Adapted from Marmer 2003.

patient's life. For example, someone who is dependent and submissive toward his or her spouse may begin to behave in that way with the analyst.

Generally, psychoanalysis is less interactive than other forms of talk psychotherapy, with the patient encouraged to say everything that comes to mind (*free association*) and the therapist listening, making comments only when, in his or her professional judgment, an opportunity for insight on the part of the patient arises. More current versions of psychoanalysis are often referred to as "insight-oriented" or "psychodynamic" psychotherapy (see the next section, "Object Relations Theory," in this chapter). These therapies have their roots in psychoanalytic theory but also borrow from other forms of psychotherapy and typically have the therapist and patient facing each other for more direct interaction. Psychoanalytic principles can also be applied to family therapy and group therapy.

Freud posited a *structural theory* of the psyche and hypothesized that many human problems resulted from unresolved conflicts among the following dimensions:

- *Id.* Contains the most primitive desires of rage (aggression) and sex (libido).
- *Superego.* Contains internalized norms, morality, and taboos.
- *Ego.* Mediates between the two and may include or give rise to the sense of self.

Resistance represents a deeply felt reluctance to bring repressed (unconscious) events or feelings to awareness. The patient may avoid memories or insights that would arouse anxiety.

Countertransference is a condition in which the therapist begins to transfer his or her own unconscious feelings to the patient. For example, a therapist may dread a psychotherapy session with a patient because the patient reminds the therapist of a negative person in the therapist's life, or a therapist may feel unusually protective of a patient who reminds the therapist of his or her own child. A well-trained therapist will use such feelings to help understand the patient.

Projective identification is a psychological process in which a patient projects a set of beliefs or emotions onto the therapist. The patient does it in such a way that the therapist begins to act as if he or she actually has the beliefs or emotions the patient projected onto the therapist. For example, a patient may feel unlikable and have low self-esteem. Initially, the therapist does not view the patient this way. However, throughout the therapy sessions, the patient behaves in such a manner as to cause the therapist to dislike him or her and to verify the patient's belief that he or she is, in fact, unlikable.

Object Relations Theory

Object relations theory is a modern adaptation of psychoanalytic theory that emphasizes human relationships as the primary motivational force in life. Object relations theorists believe that we are relationship seeking rather than pleasure seeking, as Freud suggested. The importance of relationships in the theory translates to relationships as the main focus of psychotherapy, especially the relationship with the therapist.

Psychodynamic Psychotherapy

Psychodynamic psychotherapy, also called insight-oriented psychotherapy, uses the principles of psychoanalysis but is more focused and has less frequent sessions. As opposed to classic psychoanalysis, in psychodynamic psychotherapy, the patient and therapist are seated face-to-face. The goal of treatment is for the therapist to help the patient understand and work through transference, develop insight, and improve adaptive defenses in order to resolve conflicts (Dulcan et al. 2003; Gabbard and Bennett 2007; Levenson et al. 2003).

Psychosocial Treatments

Table 15–2 summarizes the evidence-based psychosocial interventions available for major psychiatric illnesses.

Behavior Therapy

Behavior therapy is founded in the school of behaviorism, which states that psychological matters can be studied scientifically by observing overt behavior. Behavior therapy is based on the principles of classical conditioning developed by Ivan Pavlov and operant conditioning developed by B. F. Skinner (Skinner 1953). Although the theoretical underpinnings of behaviorism can be applied to almost any problem, two more comprehensive therapy techniques are particularly useful in the treatment of anxiety disorders: systematic desensitization and exposure and response prevention (ERP).

Systematic desensitization includes teaching relaxation skills in order to control fear and anxiety responses to specific phobias. Once the indi-

TABLE 15–2. Evidence-based psychosocial interventions for major psychiatric illnesses

DIAGNOSIS	INTERVENTION(S)
Any	Psychoeducation: Almost all patients can benefit from psychoeducation at varying intensities. However, for patients with active psychotic symptoms psychoeducation may be most appropriate when symptoms are stabilized or with key family or support systems.
Major depressive disorder	Cognitive-behavioral therapy (CBT) or interpersonal therapy (IPT)
Bipolar disorder	CBT, IPT (modified for bipolar disorder with an emphasis on social rhythms; this modification is called interpersonal social rhythm therapy [IPSRT]), psychoeducation, family-focused therapy
Anxiety disorders	CBT and behavior therapy
Schizophrenia	Psychoeducation if not actively psychotic, family psychoeducation
Borderline personality disorder	Dialectical behavior therapy

vidual has been taught these skills, he or she uses them to react toward and overcome situations in an established hierarchy of fears. The goal of this process is for an individual to learn to cope with and overcome the fear in each step of the hierarchy. This process will lead to overcoming the last step of the fear in the hierarchy. For example, if a person is afraid of flying, lower rungs on the hierarchy might involve imagining entering a plane or viewing pictures of airplanes. The ultimate step would be flying itself.

Exposure and response prevention is predicated on the idea that a therapeutic effect is achieved as subjects confront their fears and discontinue their escape response. An example would be of a person who repeatedly washes his or her hands after touching any foreign object. The therapy involves touching feared objects and then resisting the urge to complete the "safety behavior" (i.e., hand washing). Over time, with success in resisting the response, the patient experiences habituation to the feared stimulus.

Cognitive-Behavioral Therapy

Cognitive-behavioral therapy (CBT) is most often associated with the work of Albert Ellis and Aaron Beck, dating back to the early 1970s (Beck 1976; Beck et al. 1979; Ellis and Dryden 1987). In CBT, behaviors are thought to stem from distorted and irrational thoughts. Hence, therapy focuses on changing thoughts and behaviors directly, as opposed to trying to understand unconscious processes as in psychodynamic psychotherapy. CBT differs from behavior therapy alone because of the emphasis on assessment of distorted or irrational thoughts. Behavior therapy is only concerned with modification of observable behavior.

CBT is an active therapy that involves constant interaction between clinician and patient. Most often, it involves mutually agreed-upon goals for change, and progress toward achieving those goals is continually monitored. It often includes homework assignments between sessions, such as completing relaxation exercises or practicing assertive communication skills. The goal of CBT is for the patient to learn new skills and strategies that he or she will eventually implement independently as needed.

Interpersonal Therapy

Interpersonal psychotherapy was initially developed to treat depression (Klerman et al. 1984; Weissman et al. 2000). Stressful interpersonal events are thought to contribute to the onset of symptoms for individuals genetically prone to depression. Thus, this approach focuses on the interpersonal context in which depression symptoms emerge. Patients learn to identify problematic social patterns and relate their moods to these patterns. Clinicians help patients determine which of the following core problem areas may be contributing to their symptoms:

- *Grief over loss.*   The clinician assesses for the presence of abnormal grief. In some cases, this form of grief includes grieving over the lost "healthy" self or opportunities missed due to illness. For example, a person may grieve because he or she never finished college or may grieve for a lost relationship. Treatment focuses on facilitating the mourning process and helping the patient establish interests and relationships that can substitute for what has been lost.

- *Interpersonal conflicts.*   The patient and a significant other may have conflicting expectations about the relationship that may contribute to symptoms. Treatment goals include identifying the disputes, making choices about a plan of action, and then modifying communication patterns and/or reassessing expectations to resolve the dispute.

- *Role transitions.*   When a person has difficulty coping with life changes that require a role change, the therapist will work with the patient to give up a previous role. This includes helping the patient express anger, guilt, and loss. It may also include assistance to develop new attachments and find appropriate support groups. For example, a person may experience a divorce and have mood symptoms as a consequence of his or her dissatisfaction with life events and new status as a single person. The therapist and patient may work together to recognize the positive aspects of single life and the dissolution of an unhappy marriage. They may also work to enhance the person's social contacts and acclimate to this role change.

- *Interpersonal skills deficits.*   The interpersonal therapy model predicts that interpersonal deficits contribute to mood symptoms. Those with long histories of inadequate or superficial interpersonal relationships may have deficits that lead to social isolation. The therapist will work with the patient to reduce social isolation and acquire skills to build more intimate and lasting relationships.

Dialectical Behavior Therapy

Dialectical behavior therapy (DBT) was developed initially for use with patients with borderline personality disorder and has proven effective in decreasing self-injurious behaviors, suicide attempts, and bulimic behavior in this population (Linehan et al. 1993, 2006; Lynch et al. 2006). The dialectical nature of DBT is that it addresses both the need for acceptance and the need for change; acceptance and validation of what the patient is experiencing and change of dysfunctional thoughts, feelings, and behavior. The goal of DBT is to enhance the patient's ability to engage in functional (as opposed to dysfunctional) behavior even when experiencing intense emotions. DBT uses some techniques common to other types of therapy, such as ERP and cognitive restructuring. It also uses techniques unique to DBT, including emotion regulation and the development of distress tolerance skills.

Psychoeducation

Psychoeducation involves teaching patients and their families about their disorder, treatment options, and how to recognize signs of relapse, so they can get necessary treatment before their difficulty worsens or recurs. Additionally, those close to the patient may learn coping strategies and problem-solving skills to help them deal more effectively with the patient.

Most psychoeducational programs are integrative, with providers choosing a different focus of education depending on illness and patient characteristics. For example, if a patient demonstrates a persistent problem taking medications as prescribed, psychoeducation for that person may focus on developing tools to help the patient be more consistent (e.g., using a timer, pillbox, or medication checklist posted in a prominent location in the home). Some common psychoeducational topics include focus on taking medication as prescribed, understanding risk factors for relapse, recognizing warning signs of relapse, managing stressful life events, and learning about protective factors. For example, having daily contact with a supportive friend or attending support group meetings may be essential to sustain recovery.

Psychoeducation can be simple and straightforward (e.g., a patient and nurse discussing expected side effects of a new medication) or more complex and multifaceted (e.g., a psychoeducational "package" that may include written, visual, and interactive educational materials about the disorder and treatment). One such package was developed for use in the Texas Medication Algorithm Project (TMAP) and includes written materials, a video, pictures depicting important lessons, and instructions for an interactive, peer-led group experience. This package includes tools that provide patient and family education, address symptoms and treatment, and emphasize the development of a collaborative treatment relationship (Toprac et al. 2000). Additional program information is available at www.dshs.state.tx.us/mhprograms/TMAP.shtm.

References

Beck AT: Cognitive Therapy and the Emotional Disorders. New York, International Universities Press, 1976

Beck AT, Rush AJ, Shaw, BF, et al: Cognitive Therapy of Depression. New York, Guilford, 1979

Dulcan MK, Martini DR, Lake M: Concise Guide to Child and Adolescent Psychiatry, 3rdEdition. Washington, DC, American Psychiatric Press, 2003

Ellis A, Dryden W: The Practice of Rational-Emotive Therapy. New York, Springer, 1987

Gabbard GO, Bennett TJ: Psychodynamic psychotherapy of depression, in Gabbard's Treatment of Psychiatric Disorders. Edited by Gabbard GO. Washington, DC, American Psychiatric Publishing, 2007, pp 433–438

Klerman GL, Weissman MM, Rounsaville BJ, et al: Interpersonal Psychotherapy of Depression. New York, Basic Books, 1984

Levenson H, Butler SF, Bein E: Brief individual psychotherapy, in The American Psychiatric Publishing Textbook of Clinical Psychiatry, 4th Edition. Edited by Hales RE, Yudofsky SC. Washington, DC, American Psychiatric Publishing, 2003, pp 1151–1175

Linehan MM, Heard HL, Armstrong HE: Naturalistic follow-up of a behavioral treatment for chronically parasuicidal borderline patients. Arch Gen Psychiatry 50:971–974, 1993

Linehan MM, Comtois KA, Murray AM, et al: Two-year randomized controlled trial and follow-up of dialectical behavior therapy vs therapy by experts for suicidal behaviors and borderline personality disorder. Arch Gen Psychiatry 63:757–766, 2006

Lynch TR, Chapman AL, Rosenthal MZ, et al: Mechanisms of change in dialectical behavior therapy: theoretical and empirical observations. J Clin Psychology 62:459–480, 2006

Marmer SS: Theories of the mind and psychopathology, in The American Psychiatric Publishing Textbook of Clinical Psychiatry, 4th Edition. Edited by Hales RE, Yudofsky SC. Washington, DC, American Psychiatric Publishing, 2003, pp 107–152

Skinner BF: Science and Human Behavior. New York, Macmillan, 1953

Toprac MG, Rush AJ, Conner TM, et al: The Texas Medication Algorithm Project patient and family education program: a consumer-guided initiative. J Clin Psychiatry 61:477–486, 2000

Weissman MM, Markowitz J, Klerman GL: Comprehensive Guide to Interpersonal Psychotherapy. New York, Basic Books, 2000

16

Electroconvulsive Therapy and Device-Based Treatments

Electroconvulsive Therapy

The use of electroconvulsive therapy (ECT) was originally based on the observation that some patients with both psychosis and epilepsy were less psychotic after a seizure, hence the seizure may have been in some way "treating" the psychosis. Modern ECT is administered under general anesthesia and uses an electric current administered via electrodes placed against the skull to produce a grand mal seizure. Although the mechanism of action is unclear, ECT remains one of the most effective treatments for depression.

ECT is appropriate for the following clinical populations:

- Patients with severe major depression
- Patients with major depression with psychotic features
- Patients with mania that is not responsive to medications
- Patients with schizophrenia if there is an affective component or catatonic symptoms
- Pregnant women with severe symptoms who are in need of urgent treatment, especially for affective disorders

- Geriatric patients who are at risk because they are not eating and drinking
- Patients who have previously responded to ECT

There are no absolute contraindications to ECT. Relative contraindications include clinically significant space-occupying cerebral lesions or conditions with increased intracranial pressure, and significant cardiovascular problems, such as recent myocardial infarction, severe cardiac ischemia, and moderate to severe hypertension (including pheochromocytoma). A medical evaluation must be performed before using ECT (Table 16–1).

Anesthesia and Muscle Relaxation

Several medications are often used before and during ECT to minimize complications and discomfort associated with the treatment. Each ECT center may use a different combination. Pretreatment is often given with an anticholinergic drug such as atropine (0.4–1.0 mg intravenously [iv]) or glycopyrrolate (0.2–0.4 mg iv) to decrease the morbidity of cardiac bradyarrhythmias and aspiration.

General anesthesia is induced using a fast-acting anesthetic. Once the patient is anesthetized, intravenous succinylcholine is used for muscu-

---

TABLE 16–1.   Medical evaluation before electroconvulsive therapy

---

- Complete medical and neurological examination
- Complete blood count
- Serum electrolyte analysis
- Electrocardiogram
- Chest X ray (required because of the use of positive pressure respiration during general anesthesia)
- Evaluation by an anesthesiologist to determine risk of anesthesia
- X ray of the lumbosacral region if spinal orthopedic problems are suspected
- Computed tomography or magnetic resonance imaging of the brain if there is clinical evidence of a brain tumor or intracerebral bleeding or if there are central nervous system symptoms of uncertain etiology

lar relaxation. In general, approximately 0.5–1 mg/kg of intravenous succinylcholine is administered rapidly, immediately after the onset of general anesthesia. If there are preexisting skeletal problems or other orthopedic problems, a higher dose of succinylcholine may be required, whereas a history or evidence of pseudocholinesterase deficiency would call for a lower dose.

Once the succinylcholine is administered, the patient is ventilated with 100% oxygen until muscle fasciculations occur and motoric relaxation of the patient is accomplished. Modern ECT devices allow for simultaneous monitoring of the electroencephalogram (EEG) and electrocardiogram before, during, and after the ECT procedure. In addition, there should be frequent monitoring of blood pressure, pulse rate, and blood oxygen saturation (with pulse oximetry).

Parameters

Two major issues in the administration of the electrical stimulus include the stimulus dose and the electrode placement (i.e., placement may be nondominant unilateral or bilateral). Electrodes may be placed unilaterally on the nondominant hemisphere (i.e., over the right hemisphere for a right-handed individual and over the left hemisphere for a left-handed individual) or bilaterally. Although there have been observations that unilateral electrode placement is related to fewer cognitive side effects compared with bilateral stimulus, unilateral placement is less efficacious if comparable stimulus doses are used. However, recent studies using higher-dose unilateral ECT have demonstrated improved efficacy (Eschweiler et al. 2007; Sackeim et al. 2000).

Course of Treatment

In the United States, ECT treatments are generally given on an every-other-day basis for 2–3 weeks, usually Monday, Wednesday, and Friday. Duration of seizure for longer than 25 seconds per treatment (as assessed by motor activity, not EEG seizure activity) is considered adequate for therapeutic purposes. The number of treatments administered is generally determined by a patient's clinical response; the therapy is discontinued when successive treatments do not elicit further beneficial effects. With depressed patients, a typical course of ECT consists of 6–10 treatments, but sometimes more are required. We do not recommend more than 20 treatments in a single course of ECT.

Psychiatric Medications Affecting ECT

Some data indicate increased neurotoxicity when patients who are taking lithium receive ECT (Jha et al. 1996). Therefore, lithium should be discontinued 24 hours before ECT. Benzodiazepines and anticonvulsants increase seizure threshold, so clinicians should consider avoiding these medications within 5 half-lives when using ECT.

Risks and Side Effects

- The mortality risk is primarily related to the risk of general anesthesia.
- Ictal and postictal fluctuations in autonomic tone can elicit cardiac arrhythmias.
- The most frequent complaints of patients are short-term memory impairment and headaches.
- The initial confusion and cognitive deficits associated with ECT are usually temporary, lasting approximately 30 minutes after each treatment, and occur in most patients.
- Longer-term memory difficulty localized to the time immediately surrounding the ECT administration is frequently reported.
- Longer-term memory impairment is considered rare.
- Factors associated with an increased likelihood of memory impairment are preexisting cognitive problems, the use of bilateral electrode placement, and longer courses of treatment.
- Memory loss is greatest for public events, with less impairment in memory for autobiographical information (Lisanby et al. 2000).

Post-ECT Prophylactic Treatment

After an acute course of ECT, long-term treatment is still needed; antidepressant medications are most commonly used for this purpose. Longer-term ECT may be administered at decreasing intervals (e.g., once per week and then once per month).

Vagus Nerve Stimulation

Vagus nerve stimulation (VNS) is the first implanted device approved by the U.S. Food and Drug Administration for the treatment of a psychiatric disorder. It was approved as an adjunctive treatment for chronic and recurrent unipolar or bipolar depression nonresponsive to four adequate antidepressant treatments. The same device is used for epilepsy.

VNS should not be considered an emergency intervention; response, when it occurs, is typically delayed by 3–12 months (Rush et al. 2005). Contraindications to VNS therapy include having a history of a bilateral or left cervical vagotomy and receiving diathermy (deep-tissue heat treatment).

Method

A pacemaker-like pulse generator is surgically implanted in the left chest wall where it delivers an electrical signal through an implanted lead that is wrapped around the left cervical vagus nerve. The implanted pulse generator is then programmed with a telemetric wand using a laptop or handheld computer to deliver pulses to the vagus nerve. These are typically set for 30 seconds every 5 minutes, 24 hours a day, or until turned off.

No portion of the device is in the brain, but the intermittent stimulation of the vagus nerve produces bilateral activation of brain circuits.

Side Effects

Common side effects resulting from device stimulation of the vagus nerve are voice alteration, increased cough, dyspnea, neck pain, dysphagia, laryngismus, and paresthesias.

Transcranial Magnetic Stimulation

Transcranial magnetic stimulation (TMS) is currently investigational in the United States for treatment-resistant depression (Fitzgerald et al. 2006), but it is approved for this indication in Canada, Australia, New Zealand, the European Union, and Israel.

Method

TMS provides direct stimulation of areas of the brain believed to be involved in depression. A small coil is placed over the left frontal cortex, and the coil produces a rapidly alternating magnetic field that results in focal neuronal depolarization.

The patient remains awake during the treatment. Treatments can last 45 minutes and can occur daily. In general, patients tolerate repetitive TMS (rTMS) well and are able to resume their daily activities immediately following treatment.

Side Effects and Safety

- The most common side effects of rTMS are headache and neck pain.
- The primary safety concern with rTMS is seizures.

Deep Brain Stimulation

Deep brain stimulation (DBS) is investigational for significantly treatment-resistant depression and obsessive-compulsive disorder (Greenberg et al. 2006; Mayberg et al. 2005).

Method

The device consists of an implantable battery-powered pulse generator (IPG) implanted near the clavicle similar to pacemakers or VNS devices. One or two leads (unilateral or bilateral) are tunneled from the device(s) under the scalp along the skull. Neuroimaging and brain stimulation recording during the implantation procedure facilitate exact placement of the lead in the targeted brain area. The anatomic target of DBS differs depending on the underlying disease, and even with the same disease there is ongoing debate about optimal targets.

Side Effects

The most common side effects are from the procedure itself. These include infection, skin erosion, subcutaneous seroma, and intercerebral hematoma.

References

Eschweiler GW, Vonthein R, Bode R, et al: Clinical efficacy and cognitive side effects of bifrontal versus right unilateral electroconvulsive therapy (ECT): a short term randomized controlled trial in pharmaco-resistant major depression. J Affect Disorders 101:149–157, 2007

Fitzgerald PB, Benitez J, De Castella A, et al: A randomized, controlled trial of sequential bilateral repetitive transcranial magnetic stimulation for treatment-resistant depression. Am J Psychiatry 163:88–94, 2006

Greenberg BD, Malone DA, Friehs GM, et al: Three-year outcomes in deep brain stimulation for highly resistant obsessive-compulsive disorder. Neuropsychopharmacology 31:2384–2393, 2006

Jha AK, Stein GS, Fenwick P: Negative interaction between lithium and electroconvulsive therapy—a case-control study. Br J Psychiatry 168:241–243, 1996

Lisanby SH, Maddox JH, Prudic J, et al: The effects of electroconvulsive therapy on memory of autobiographical and public events. Arch Gen Psychiatry 57:581–590, 2000

Mayberg HS, Lozano AM, Voon V, et al: Deep brain stimulation for treatment-resistant depression. Neuron 45:651–660, 2005

Rush AJ, Sackeim HA, Marangell LB, et al: Effects of 12 months of vagus nerve stimulation in treatment-resistant depression: a naturalistic study. Biol Psychiatry 58:355–363, 2005

Sackeim HA, Prudic J, Devanand DP, et al: A prospective, randomized, double-blind comparison of bilateral and right unilateral electroconvulsive therapy at different stimulus intensities. Arch Gen Psychiatry 57:425–434, 2000

Appendix 1

Commonly Used Abbreviations

AA Alcoholics Anonymous

AABH Association for Ambulatory Behavioral Healthcare

AACAP American Academy of Child and Adolescent Psychiatry

AAEP American Association of Emergency Psychiatry

AAIDD American Association on Intellectual and Developmental Disabilities

AAMC Association of American Medical Colleges

AAMI age-associated memory impairment

AAN American Academy of Neurology

AAPDP American Academy of Psychoanalysis and Dynamic Psychiatry

AAPL American Academy of Psychiatry and the Law

ABMS American Board of Medical Specialties

ABPN American Board of Psychiatry and Neurology

ACNP American College of Neuropsychopharmacology

ACOPSA   American College of Psychoanalysts

ACP   American College of Physicians; American College of Psychiatrists; Association for Child Psychoanalysis

ACTH   adrenocorticotropic hormone

AD   Alzheimer's disease

ADD   attention-deficit disorder

ADH   alcohol dehydrogenase

ADHD   attention-deficit/hyperactivity disorder

ADMSEP   Association of Directors of Medical Student Education in Psychiatry

ADR   acute dystonic reaction

AFMR   American Federation for Medical Research

AFSP   American Foundation for Suicide Prevention

AFTA   American Family Therapy Academy

AGPA   American Group Psychotherapy Association

AIDS   acquired immunodeficiency syndrome

AIMS   Abnormal Involuntary Movement Scale

AIPP   American Institute for Psychotherapy and Psychoanalysis

AJP   American Journal of Psychiatry

ALS   amyotrophic lateral sclerosis

ALT   alanine aminotransferase (alanine transaminase)

AMA   against medical advice; American Medical Association

AMHA   American Mental Health Alliance

AMSA   American Medical Student Association

ANA   antinuclear antibody

ANAD   National Association of Anorexia Nervosa and Associated Disorders

ANS   autonomic nervous system

AOA   American Orthopsychiatric Association

APA   American Psychiatric Association; American Psychological Association

APC   Association of Professional Chaplains

APM   Academy of Psychosomatic Medicine

APPI   American Psychiatric Publishing, Inc.

APsaA   American Psychoanalytic Association

ASAM   American Society of Addiction Medicine

ASLME   American Society of Law, Medicine and Ethics

AWA   away without authorization

BDD   body dysmorphic disorder

BEAM   brain electrical activity mapping

bid   twice a day

BIS   Brain Information Service

BMA   British Medical Association

BMI   body mass index

BPD   borderline personality disorder

BUN   blood urea nitrogen

CA   Cocaine Anonymous

CAT   Children's Apperception Test

CBC   complete blood count

CBT   cognitive-behavioral therapy

CISD   critical incident stress debriefing

CME   continuing medical education

CMHC   community mental health center

CNS   central nervous system

CPT   Current Procedural Terminology (AMA); cognitive processing therapy

CRF   corticotropin-releasing factor

CSF   cerebrospinal fluid

CT   computed tomography

CVA   cerebrovascular accident; stroke

DBH   dopamine β-hydroxylase

DBS   deep brain stimulation

DBSA   Depression and Bipolar Support Alliance

DBT   dialectical behavior therapy

DHHS   U.S. Department of Health and Human Services

DID   dissociative identity disorder

DNA   deoxyribonucleic acid

DOV   discharged on visit

DRG   diagnosis-related group

DSM   *Diagnostic and Statistical Manual of Mental Disorders*

DST   dexamethasone suppression test

DTs   delirium tremens

EA   Emotions Anonymous

EAP   employee assistance program

ECA   Epidemiologic Catchment Area

ECG   electrocardiogram

ECT   electroconvulsive therapy

EE   expressed emotion

EEG   electroencephalogram

EKG   electrocardiogram (ECG is preferred abbreviation)

EMDR   eye movement desensitization and reprocessing

EMG   electromyogram

ESP   extrasensory perception

EST   electroshock treatment

FDA   U.S. Food and Drug Administration

GA   Gamblers Anonymous

GABA γ-aminobutyric acid

GAF   Global Assessment of Functioning

GAP   Group for the Advancement of Psychiatry

GHB   γ-hydroxybutyric acid

GSR   galvanic skin response

Ham-D   Hamilton Rating Scale for Depression (also HRSD)

HIPAA   Health Insurance Portability and Accountability Act

HIV   human immunodeficiency virus

HMO   health maintenance organization

HRSD   Hamilton Rating Scale for Depression (also Ham-D)

ICD   International Classification of Diseases

ICSW   International Council on Social Welfare

IND   investigational new drug

IOM/NAS   Institute of Medicine/National Academy of Sciences

IPT   interpersonal (psycho)therapy

IQ   intelligence quotient

ITAA   International Transactional Analysis Association

IV   intravenous(ly)

JCAHO   Joint Commission on Accreditation of Healthcare Organizations (name changed to The Joint Commission in 2007)

LP   lumbar puncture

LSD   lysergic acid diethylamide

MA   mental age

MAO   monoamine oxidase

MAOI   monoamine oxidase inhibitor

MBD   minimal brain dysfunction

MDI   manic-depressive illness

MDMA   3,4-methylenedioxymethamphetamine (Ecstasy)

MET   motivational enhancement therapy

MHA   Mental Health Association

MMPI   Minnesota Multiphasic Personality Inventory

MMSE   Mini-Mental State Examination

MRAA   Mental Retardation Association of America

MRI   magnetic resonance imaging

MSE   mental status examination

NA   Narcotics Anonymous

NAMI   National Alliance on Mental Illness

NARSAD   National Alliance for Research on Schizophrenia and Depression

NAS   National Academy of Sciences

NBME   National Board of Medical Examiners

NCADD   National Council on Alcoholism and Drug Dependence

NCCBH   National Council for Community Behavioral Healthcare (formerly National Council of Community Mental Health Centers)

NCS   National Comorbidity Study; National Comorbidity Survey

NCSE   Neurobehavioral Cognitive Status Examination

NIA   National Institute on Aging

NIAAA   National Institute on Alcohol Abuse and Alcoholism

NIDA   National Institute on Drug Abuse

NIH   National Institutes of Health

NIMH   National Institute of Mental Health

NMA   National Medical Association

NMDA   N-methyl-D-aspartate

NMR   nuclear magnetic resonance

NMS   neuroleptic malignant syndrome

NOS   not otherwise specified

NREM   non–rapid eye movement

NSF   National Science Foundation

OCD   obsessive-compulsive disorder

PCP   phencyclidine

PDD   pervasive developmental disorder

PDR   *Physicians' Desk Reference*

PET   positron emission tomography

PKU   phenylketonuria

PRO   peer review organization

PSRO   professional standards review organization

PTSD   posttraumatic stress disorder

qid   four times a day

rCBF   regional cerebral blood flow

REM   rapid eye movement

RNA   ribonucleic acid

SAD   seasonal affective disorder

SAMHSA   Substance Abuse and Mental Health Services Administration

SCID-I   Structured Clinical Interview for DSM-IV Axis I Disorders

SDA   serotonin-dopamine antagonist

SDAT   senile dementia of the Alzheimer's type

SNRI   serotonin-norepinephrine reuptake inhibitor

SOBP   Society of Biological Psychiatry

SPECT   single photon emission computed tomography

SPEM   smooth pursuit eye movement

SSI/SSDI   Social Security Insurance/Social Security Disability Insurance

SSRI   selective serotonin reuptake inhibitor

TIA   transient ischemic attack

tid   three times a day

TM   transcendental meditation

TMS   transcranial magnetic stimulation

TRH   thyrotropin-releasing hormone

USPHS   U.S. Public Health Service

VA   Veterans Affairs (formerly Veterans Administration)

VCFS   velocardiofacial syndrome

VDRL   Venereal Disease Research Laboratory

VNS   vagus nerve stimulation

WHO   World Health Organization

WMA   World Medical Association

WPA   World Psychiatric Association

Trade/Brand Names of Common Psychiatric Drugs

TABLE 18–1.

GENERIC	TRADE/BRAND NAME
Alprazolam	Xanax
Amantadine	Symadine, Symmetrel
Amitriptyline	Elavil, Endep, Enovil
Amitriptyline/perphenazine	Triavil
Amphetamine/dextroamphetamine	Adderall
Amoxapine	Asendin
Aripiprazole	Abilify
Benztropine	Cogentin
Bromocriptine	Parlodel
Bupropion	Wellbutrin
Buspirone	BuSpar
Carbamazepine	Epitol, Tegretol
Chlordiazepoxide	Librium, Libritabs
Chlorpromazine	Ormazine, Thorazine

TABLE 18–1.

GENERIC	TRADE/BRAND NAME
Citalopram	Celexa
Clomipramine	Anafranil
Clonazepam	Klonopin
Clorazepate	Tranxene
Clozapine	Clozaril
Cyproheptadine	Periactin
Dantrolene	Dantrium
Desipramine	Norpramin, Pertofrane
Dexmethylphenidate	Focalin
Desmethylvenlafaxine	Pristiq
Dextroamphetamine	Dexedrine, Dextrostat
Diazepam	Valium
Diphenhydramine	Benadryl
Divalproex	Depakote
Donepezil	Aricept
Doxepin	Adapin, Sinequan
Duloxetine	Cymbalta
Escitalopram	Lexapro
Estazolam	ProSom
Eszopiclone	Lunesta
Fluoxetine	Prozac
Fluphenazine	Prolixin
Fluvoxamine	Luvox
Gabapentin	Neurontin

TABLE 18–1.

GENERIC	TRADE/BRAND NAME
Galantamine	Reminyl
Haloperidol	Haldol
Hydroxyzine	Atarax, Marax, Vistaril
Imipramine	Tofranil
Isocarboxazid	Marplan
Lamotrigine	Lamictal
Levetiracetam	Keppra
Lithium	Eskalith, Lithobid
Lorazepam	Ativan
Loxapine	Loxitane
Maprotiline	Ludiomil
Mesoridazine	Serentil
Methylphenidate	Concerta, Metadate, Methylin, Ritalin
Mexiletine	Mexitil
Midazolam	Versed
Mirtazapine	Remeron
Moclobemide	Aurorix
Modafinil	Provigil, Alertec
Molindone	Moban
Naloxone	Narcan
Naltrexone	ReVia
Nefazodone	Serzone

TABLE 18–1.

GENERIC	TRADE/BRAND NAME
Nifedipine	Adalat
Nortriptyline	Aventyl, Pamelor
Olanzapine	Zyprexa
Oxazepam	Serax
Oxcarbazepine	Trileptal
Paroxetine	Paxil
Pargyline	Eutonyl
Pemoline	Cylert
Perphenazine	Etrafon, Trilafon
Phenelzine	Nardil
Phenytoin	Dilantin
Physostigmine	Eserine
Pimozide	Orap
Pindolol	Visken
Pramipexole	Mirapex
Propranolol	Inderal
Protriptyline	Vivactil
Quazepam	Doral, Dormalin
Quetiapine	Seroquel
Ramelteon	Rozerem
Risperidone	Risperdal
Rivastigmine	Exelon
Selegiline, L-deprenyl	Carbex, Eldepryl

TABLE 18–1.

GENERIC	TRADE/BRAND NAME
Sertraline	Zoloft
Sildenafil	Viagra
Tacrine	Cognex
Temazepam	Restoril
Thioridazine	Mellaril
Thiothixene	Navane
Thyroxine	Synthroid
Tianeptine	Stablon
Topiramate	Topamax
Tranylcypromine	Parnate
Trazodone	Desyrel
Triazolam	Halcion
Trifluoperazine	Stelazine
Triflupromazine	Vesprin
Trihexyphenidyl	Artane
Triiodothyronine	Cytomel
Trimipramine	Surmontil
Valproate	Depakene, Depakote
Venlafaxine	Effexor
Verapamil	Calan, Isoptin
Zaleplon	Sonata
Ziprasidone	Geodon
Zolpidem	Ambien
Zonisamide	Zonegran

Index

*Page numbers printed in **boldface** type refer to tables or figures.*

NOTES

NOTES

NOTES

NOTES

NOTES

NOTES